PRIMARY HEALTH CARE AND REFUGEES

Primary Health Care Publications

General Editor:

Prof.dr. Ivan Wolffers
Department of Social Medicine
Vrije Universiteit
Van der Boechorststraat 7
1081 BT Amsterdam
the Netherlands

Published in this series:

1. Patients without frontiers
Ivan Wolffers
90-6256-937-4 [1990] 72 pages ppb

2. The role of traditional medicine in primary health care
Ivan Wolffers (ed.)
90-6256-936-6 [1990] 80 pages ppb

3. Primary health care and diarrhoea
Ivan Wolffers and Daniel Nelson (eds.)
90-5383-042-1 [1991] 88 pages ppb

4. AIDS and primary health care
Ivan Wolffers (ed.)
90-5383-043-x [1992] 84 pages ppb

5. Health in Bangladesh
Ivan Wolffers
90-5383-146-0 [1992] 116 pages ppb

6. The impact of injections in daily medical practice
Maurice Bloem and Ivan Wolffers (eds.)
90-5383-147-9 [1993] 140 pages ppb

7. The handicapped community
Harry Finkenflügel (ed.)
90-5383-211-4 [1993] 160 pages ppb

8. Altering the image of AIDS
Maria de Bruyn (ed.)
90-5383-259-9 [1994] 136 pages ppb

9. Primary health care and refugees
Anke van der Kwaak and Ivan Wolffers (eds.)
90-5383-333-1 [1996] 114 pages ppb

10. Health and health care in transition
Eric Naterop and Ivan Wolffers (eds.)
90-5383-406-0 [1995] 116 pages ppb

PRIMARY HEALTH CARE AND REFUGEES

Anke van der Kwaak and Ivan Wolffers (eds.)

VU University Press
Amsterdam 1996

The series Primary Health Care Publications is a platform for scholars and practitioners to share their research and their fieldwork experiences.
If you are interested in translating and/or adapting this book, please contact the address below. We will be pleased to assist you in this matter.

Prof.dr. Ivan Wolffers
Department of Social Medicine
Vrije Universiteit
Van der Boechorststraat 7
1081 BT Amsterdam
the Netherlands

VU University Press is an imprint of:
VU Boekhandel/Uitgeverij bv
De Boelelaan 1105
1081 HV Amsterdam
the Netherlands

issn 0926-9827
isbn 90-5383-333-1
nugi 732

cover: D PS, Amsterdam
cover photo: Md. Mainuddin, (Dhaka) Bangladesh

CONTENTS **page**

PREFACE

This is the ninth volume in the Primary Health Care Publication series. This contribution gives an overview of some recent developments with regard to international migration and refugee matters.

In a world where living conditions in some parts are unbearable because of violence, environmental degradation or lack of economic perspectives, more and more people decide to look for better places to live. Some are permanent emigrants, some are temporary ones. In some situations the flow of people is acute and massive. This is especially the case in parts of the world where the emergency sitiation is acute. These people, among whom often many women and unaccompanied children, end up in refugee camps and are not always prepared for the new situation. Nor are the health care workers that deal with the problems of refugees.

In this publication contributions have been brought together of people who have been working in the field of refugees and health, like Anica Kos, Annemiek Richters, Loes van Willigen, Jeanette Lekskes, Marijke Wijnroks, Ivan Wolffers and Anke van der Kwaak. The objective behind this publication is both to stimulate discussion on structural health care for refugees and displaced people versus more temporary forms of aid, relief and rehabilitation. Also violence against women will be discussed. The contributions in this volume give examples of the former Yugoslavia, Africa, the Netherlands and Bangladesh in order to give those interested in other parts of the world to learn from these various experiences described.

This publication (like all others in this series) can be translated and adapted to local circumstances to educate and create awareness. In addition, we invite those who desire to set up activities like surveys, educational programmes, workshops, or those who wish more information to contact the *Department of Social Medicine, Section Health Care in Developing Countries, Van der Boechorststraat 7, 1081 BT Amsterdam*.

In preparing this publication, we have been helped and encouraged by many people. We would like to thank the authors for their contribution, and Ms Patricia Brinckman who kindly assisted us with the index and lay-out.

Anke van der Kwaak
Ivan Wolffers

Amsterdam, December 1995

1. INTRODUCTION. HEALTH AND CONFLICT SITUATIONS: FROM EMERGENCY AID TO SUSTAINABLE DEVELOPMENT

Anke van der Kwaak en Ivan Wolffers

Introduction

Uwimbabazi Pascazliya is fourteen years old and living in an orphanage in Rwanda. During the fightings of one and half year ago she and her parents found refuge in a church. But some youngsters came, carrying chopping knives and cudgels. Her brothers, sisters and parents died. She and her brother pretended to be dead and survived the slaughtering. They fled, but again were found by militias, and her brother was literally cut into pieces. Uwimbabazi arrived traumatised in the orphanage of Kabgayi in Rwanda. She is one of the more than 400.000 traumatised unaccompanied children living in orphanages in Rwanda. A national programma is needed not only for them but also for the social workers who are traumatised themselves. Also children of the people responsible for the slaughtering are severely traumatised. Leslie McTyre psycho-social working for UNICEF in Rwanda says it in this way: "the vicious circle in which the children who grow up with violence and conflict has to be broken down, otherwise as adults, they will solve any problem with chopping knives"[1].

This shocking story is only one of the many cases in which violence and war cause the displacement of people. At this moment of time, while we are heading towards the end of the twentieth century, refugees and displaced people form a fast growing population in the world. Around 25 million people have fled their homes, their villages, their regions or their countries. Often, as in the case of Uwimbabazi, they are haunted by military or rebel groups, or by government armies for reasons of ethnicity, religion, war and violence. Others have sought other places where they themselves and their families have better chances for survival.

This book focuses on refugees and health in the broadest sense. Uwimbabazi has found refuge in an orphanage in Rwanda itself, while many others have travelled

across borders. Their mental and psychical health are at stake. How can we support systems to be developed to help children like Uwimbabazi to cope with such situations? Do we need more volunteers who rush to the areas in crisis to amputate legs or console orphaned children, while in addition they inform those watching news-programmes at home that something has to be done? Or is it possible to develop structural programmes to prevent this kind of disasters, and empower refugees to cope with their new situation?
Often people only seem to think about the possibility of emergency aid, but this books shows that creative structural support is quite well possible. Ideas like they are embedded in the primary health care strategy seem to be useful for that. This can be organized in the country of conflict, in the first country where people seek refuge or in the country where the refugees finally end up. In all these situations, the recipe is the same: empower them instead of making them dependent of the benevolence of donors or enemies. However, do we want refugees to be empowered?
In this book we like to explore the ways in which can be best dealt with refugee situations in terms of health. Before we will introduce the contributions, some definitions should be cleared and the causes of emergencies and answers to that in terms of development aid are to be discussed.

Refugees

90% of the refugees in the world, stay in the surroundings of their own region or country[2]. This means that the countries and regions people fly from are mainly in the South. Because of the recent refugee flows from Former-Yugoslavia and Eastern Europe, Europe received in 1993 26.3% refugees, while Africa exceeds this number by 32.8%. Croatia, with a population of 2 million has received around 600,000 refugees from Bosnia-Herzegovina and Serbs from occupied territories[3].
These numbers throw another light on the debate in Northern countries on how to stop the massive flow of refugees. In the Netherlands, for example, the idea exists that the country is full and has reached the limits of population growth, while in reality most refugees find refuge in their own regions.

At this moment of time, the Dutch government has decided that greater parts of e.g. Somalia and Sri Lanka are so called 'safe areas' were refugees can be sent back to.

Because refugees' problems are more and more formulated as problems of receiving countries the policies to deal with refugees (who are also the main donors) have changed overtime. Policies nowadays stress temporary stay in the host country and less structural programmes to integrate newcomers. They give support to emergency aid in neighbouring countries of countries in conflict in order to keep refugees there, which is at the cost of structural aid of the region. This may play a modest role in preventing the conditions that create violence and make people decide to migrate to safer areas or places where they have less trouble to survive.

Like many other countries in the world, the Dutch system of right of asylum is based on the Convention of Geneva of 1951[4], The Convention was originally designed for Post-War Europe, but this limitation in time and geographical border was phased out by The UN Protocol of 1967. The Convention is still quite limited in its definition of refugees, but on ground of Article 33 of the Convention refugees can not be sent back to their countries as long as they fear for prosecution when returning.

Nowadays, we not only distinguish among refugees according to the Convention, but also 'displaced', 'tolerated', 'illegal', 'undocumented' persons, 'economical refugees', 'migrants' and 'asylum-seekers' have entered the refugee arena. Before the concept of migration was only used for labour migration, but nowadays 'migration' is also used for refugee flows. A recent report put it in this way: "the description of concepts doesn't take root any more; migrants become refugees (for example former Yugoslavian labour migrants in Europe), and on their turn refugees sometimes become migrants (Vietnamese boat refugees in Western countries)". The distinction among voluntary or non-voluntary refugees seems in many cases meaningless. People coming from developing countries, flee in large groups, sometimes across borders (Somalia, Rwanda, Surinam), sometimes not. In terms of the Convention only those people who have actually crossed borders are true refugees. That means that neither muslim refugees inside the former Yugoslavia, nor children like Umwimbababzi and those refugees forced to move by natural disasters and famine are seen as refugees[5].

The United Nations Higher Commissioner for Refugees (UNHCR) aims at the protection of refugees in the sense that the rights of refugees has to be broadened and safeguarded, as well as the security of refugees themselves, international action and jurisprudence. The criteria for defining which people fall under the UNHCR mandate are: prosecution, violence or conflict about political, religious, ethnic, racial or social reasons. forced departure abroad caused by these factors, and the extent to which they need protection[6]. In practice also people who have fled inside their countries like Somali's or former-Yugoslavians can get as individual cases protection from the UNHCR.

In this book the focus will be on refugees in the widest sense: not only those people who have crossed borders, but also those who are forced to leave their homes because of famine, war, fear or other reasons are defined as refugees. Included will be also people who are in the process of asking political asylum in western or other countries, but did not get an official refugee status or were refused as such in one way or the other. The question that remains unanswered is which situations cause the displacement of people and refugee flows.

Causes of emergency situations

Often a distinction is made among 4 types of emergency situations, namely, rapid onset emergencies such as natural disasters, floods and earthquakes. Secondly, slow onset emergencies such as droughts, and consequent crop failure and loss of livestock. Third, permanent emergencies such as structural poverty, economic, social and political marginalisation, and exacerbated natural disasters. And, fourth complex political emergencies such as internal political wars[7]. This four types are of course interrelated and mainly developed for Africa. Such a classification helps by defining where refugees come from, and in which respect they are traumatised, and maybe by the defining of the structure of the aid intervention following on it. But it also obscures power relations, and political structures. What is an omission here, is that complex political emergencies are often not caused by internal problems only, but also by colonial interventions, and globalisation effects. A historical dimension in looking at countries and societies is essential for really judging the future emergency situation in its value. Two concepts used within thinking about emergency situations are 'vulnerability' on the one hand, and 'protection' at the other hand. Vulnerability is used in terms of physical, social and psychological vulnerability. Physical stands for ecological and economical deprivation, social stands for social and political marginalisation, and psychological vulnerability stands for the victimisation and mental disabilities to cope with emergency situations[8].

'Protection' as a concept is especially used by the UNHCR. It is one of the aims of the work of UNHCR in order to safeguard the vulnerability of refugees in terms of physical, social and sexual vulnerability. They support their programmes by listing and distinguishing among sorts of violations and emergency situations, and the development of guidelines e.g. on sexual violence against women.

Prevention of conflict situations

What is of interest here, is that only in the last years the discussion has been started about the use of emergency aid, the assumptions underlying it, and what can be done to prevent conflict situations. Often it seems to be forgotten that in case of education and consciousness raising with respect to changing behaviour, 4 conditions are to be met, namely people must know how, they must want it, they must be able to change, and they must be allowed to change their behaviour[9].

At the moment 185 countries in the world are engaged in conflict situations. When conflicts occur two actions seem to take place: military UN-interventions and/or humanitarian (emergency) aid. Both actions seem to focus on governments, military leaders or warlords only, while also in terms of the humanitarian aid, the needs and ideas of the civil society itself are left out and not heard. Of course, one can say, who is this civil society ? Are not they as guilty as everyone else? Nowadays, we have seen how civil wars disrupt local structures on the one hand, and as a result of UN-interventions the different fighting parties involved only become more polarized than they were before. Local NGOs and civil society itself have to be supported, in a sense that the ideas of local people not belonging to governments or military groups have to be taken into account before it is to late.

A world-wide discussion is going on concerning the invention of early-warning systems, in which NGOs and not the UN - for a change - has a major role to play. In the Netherlands NGOs are making an effort in joining hands in the prevention of conflict situations. They made recommendations to the Dutch government which included the use of local NGOs, preventive diplomacy, media information, and training and research[10].

Initiatives like this one must be granted. Many humanitarian organisations are in a state of crises. They feel that they have become part of genocides, and that they involuntary support people who are slaughtering others. Most humanitarian organisations seem to remain neutral while or do they have to fulfil their jobs along with military partners, and almost have to buy themselves into countries and conflict-situations. The Rwandan Jean-Marie Vianney Bemeke who coordinates 200 local NGOs in Rwanda described the hundreds of emergency-relief organisations coming to him offering money as follows: "The humanitarian organisations look like moths coming to the lights of camera's"[11].

Violence

An important issue to be mentioned in this respect, is the fact that refugees can be considered as victims of so called 'organized violence'. This comprises any violence action which is unaccepted by human standards, and related to the victims feelings. Organized violence includes torture, cruel inhuman or degrading treatment or imprisonment without trial, mock execution, hostage taking or any other form of violent deprivation[12]. Violence against women in this respect concerns 'any act of gender-based violence that results in, or is likely to result in, physical, sexual and psychological harm or suffering to women, including threats of such acts, coercion, arbitrary deprivations of liberty, whether occurring in public or private'[13]. It was not so long ago when a representative of Amnesty International in London mentioned the reports on massive rape of women a hysteria of the media. Nowadays, also Amnesty International makes another stand, and points at rape as an instrument of war and distorted power relations.
In Kenya's North Eastern Province hundreds of women have been reported to be raped in 1992-1993. UNHCR documented 192 cases of rape, of which 187 involved women, 4 against children and one was against a man[14]. A Somali UNHCR consultant conducted research in the camps, and came up with actions and interventions e.g. counselling services, medical referral possibilities, physical protection measures, transfer to other camps, replacement of cloths and looted items, and training courses for camp officials and policemen[15]. As a result of the fact that violence of women is a global problem, the UNHCR designed useful guidelines on preventing and responding to sexual violence for field workers and others working in the refugee context[16].

What is of importance here, is that with respect to sexual violence one is about to leave the traditional emergency relief arena, and one has to think about taking preventive measures, such as looking into cultural issues when designing a refugee camp, and in case of counselling taking so called traditional coping mechanism as a starting point. New initiatives have to be mentioned here such as 'Arms to fight, arms to protect. Women speak out about conflict'. In this book, testimonies of women all-around the world are given expressing their views on conflict. From their individual stories the general picture becomes clear that also women must be heard and seen in the context of conflict and violence, and not only brought under the category of 'victimised women and children'[17].

Conflict and health

What does this all mean for the health and the well-being of people? Armed conflicts but also other forms of suppression have an enormous impact on the physical and mental health of people. The thousands of traumatised children in Rwanda is only one of the examples. Will it be enough when they are going to be counselled and trained in coping with the terror they have seen in front of their eyes? There is an international call for 'truth and justice' before the healing process can start. Some are convinced that only an international tribunal can start the healing process. Only after truth and justice, reconciliation and forgiveness can start[18].

What at least comes out from discussion like this, is that the current direction of humanitarian aid, might not be the best one. It seems that after the first emergency aid has been provided for, and the people in question are safe, whether that is in their own environment, in another country or even at another continent, a process has to start in which the people involved are not made apathetic dependent actors within semi-temporary structures, but instead they should be allowed to come up with their own ideas, views or feelings. And if that is not possible, one has to look through counselling and training into the dynamics of their former life. The fact that many asylum-seekers in the Netherlands can survive in terms of 'bed, bread and bath', shows that their abilities to work, clean, study or what so ever are not taken serious.

Self-reliance and community participation the ideals of Primary Health Care, seem to be long forgotten in emergency- and conflict situations. But recently world-wide new initiatives have come to the fore. An example to be mentioned here is the work by the Danish International Rehabilitation Council for Torture Victims (IRCT) and their project 'Treatment and Rehabilitation of victims of Multiple Trauma and rape in Bosnia-Herzegovina'. The director of this project Libby Tata Arcel chose to support local professionals and organisations. Their psycho-social project is described in a publication, in which also the characteristics/conditions of this project are made clear: namely the establishment of a local NGO, the project is community-based, the empowerment of local professionals and non-professionals is a central issue, the collaborators must be without cultural prejudices, the organization must be cultural sensitive, a separate project for raped women, has been started and in general one aims at the avoidance of pathologization; "refugees and displace people are psychologically traumatised, but not psychologically disturbed!"[19.]

Health programmes for refugees are often introduced from outside the country by medical or technical people that are often not community development people. They often have a relief orientation, get funds for medical assistance, not for preventive health care programmes. The health system to be created is not often a part of the regular health care programme. In Somalia Memisa, a Dutch NGO arranged emergency aid in a different way. It funded a regional health project where also returned refugees profited from. They funded and renewed the old hospital structure while at the same time the out-reach preventive programme was started. The work was done by Somali nationals who were trained with the help and technical assistance by 4-6 Dutch medical volunteers. This project has been closed because of political reasons, but nevertheless it tells us that the most important question remains what PHC can mean for refugee health, and what can be done in terms of community participation and self-reliance in refugee situations.

About this book

All this demonstrates the necessity for more an in-depth discussion about relief, aid and assistance to displaced people, refugees and other victims of organized violence. In this book the contributions offered, show interesting and useful examples for this discussion.

Anica Mikus Kos, a child psychiatrist, takes us to the world of refugee children in Slovenia, and she gives us a challenging approach of how that well-being of these children best can be guarded. She describes extensively how mental health activities were creatively integrated into school systems, and how the mental health team worked with primary schools.

Annemiek Richters, who holds a chair in women's health care in the Netherlands, points at what type of linkages between human rights and development are most favourable for the protection of women's right to freedom from gender violence. In her contribution, she not only mentions guidelines in this context, but she also underlines the role of health workers, the identification of invisible wounds, and how to support healing efforts by participatory research and counselling.

Marijke Wijnroks, a medical doctor working as a technical advisor in community based health care situations, describes in her contribution how Rohingyas, a Muslim ethnic minority group in Burma, entered Bangladesh, and ended up in a 'better' situation than the local population. This fact even resulted in violent clashes between refugees and local inhabitants. This subject is difficult to discuss in ethical terms, but a very real problem when we are looking today at similar problems in Tanzania and Zaire.

Jeanette Lekskes, a teacher nurse, shares her experience in participatory training or refugees as Community Workers in Hagdera Camp, Kenya with us. She convinces us that refugees should be trained as CHWs in a participatory way, whereby refugees establish services according to their needs.

Loes van Willigen ends this book with a contribution in which a public health perspective is offered on health care for refugees and asylum-seekers in the Netherlands. As the Director of the Pharos Foundation for Refugee Health, she observes how the current Dutch restrictive measures endanger prevention and health promotion activities of asylum-seekers. Her article is especially of interest for those who are not aware of the short-comings of the European system. Also here major steps has to be taken, before sustainable assistance can be given to refugees who have experienced terror and fear like Uwimbabazi Pascazliya.

References

1. Free translated and summarized from Bengt van Loosdrecht. Het ergste is, dat ik mijn broertje niet heb gered. Rwandas kinderen moeten over hun ervaringen leren praten. *Internationale Samenwerking. 12, 1994. pp. 30 -32.*
2. Ruud Huurman. Het probleem van de toekomst. *Rode Kruis Koerier. Themanummer: Vluchtelingen. 55e jaargang nr. 6, December 1994. pp. 6-8.*
3. Refugees worldwide in 1994:

Africa	7.45 million
Asia	5.77 million
Europe	6.05 million
Latin-America	0.13 million
USA	1.29 million
Oceanie	0.05 million
Former Soviet-Union	2.28 million

Source: Ruud Huurman. Het probleem van de toekomst. *ibid*. p. 7.

4. This act has been revised by the Protocol of the Status of Refugees of New York, 1967 which sounds:
" any person who owing to well-found fear of being persecuted for reasons of race, religion, nationality, membership of a particular social group or political opinion, is outside the country of its nationality and is unable or, owing to such fear unwilling to avail himself of the protection of that country; or who, not having a nationality and being outside of the country of his former habitual residence is unable or owing to such fear is unwilling to return to it".
5. Nationale Adviesraad voor Ontwikkelingssamenwerking. *Advies Vluchtelingen, Ontheemden en Ontwikkelingssamenwerking*. Den Haag: NAR. 1993, p. 9.
6. Nationale Adviesraad voor Ontwikkelingssamenwerking, Advies Vluchtelingen. *ibid*. p. 11.
7. Dutch Interchurch Aid (DIA) & Interchurch Organization for development Cooperation (ICCO). *Working document on relief, rehabilitation and development in Africa. Guidelines for policies and practices of DIA, ICCO, Churches and NGOs*. Utrecht/Zeist: DIA & ICCO. 1994. p. 7.
8. Dutch Interchurch Aid (DIA) & Interchurch Organization for development Cooperation (ICCO). *ibid*. p. 8.

9. Nommensen, Eline, *Oorlogsslachtoffers in Ethiopië & voorlichting.* Unpublished paper for the Department of Social Medicine, Free University of Amsterdam. May 1995.
10. *Uitstel wordt duur betaald, Een Notitie van het Nederlands NGO-Overleg over de Preventie van Conflictescalatie met Aanbevelingen voor de Nederlandse Regering.* Amsterdam: NCO. Maart 1995.
11. Offenberg, Willem. 'Supermarkt zonder supervisie'. Failliet humanitaire hulp lijkt in zicht. *Wordt Vervolgd. nr.10, October 1995.* pp. 4-6.
12. Van Willigen, L.H.M. & A.J.K. Hondius, *Vluchtelingen en gezondheid - theoretische beschouwingen.* Amsterdam: Swets & Zeitlinger. 1992.
13. Richters, Annemiek J.M., *Women, Culture and Violence.* A development, health and human rights issue. Women and Autonomy Series. Leiden: VENA. 1994. p. 2.
14. Africa Watch Women's Rights Project, *Seeking refuge, finding terror.* The widespread rape of Somali women refugees in North Eastern Kenya, October 4, 1993. Vol. 5. no. 13.
15. Musse, Fouzia. *Women victims of Violence. Report on Refugee camps in Kenya,* Nairobi: UNHCR. October 15, 1993.
16. UNHCR. Sexual violence against refugees. Guidelines on Prevention and response. Geneva: UNHCR. 1995.
17. Bennet, Olivia, Jo Bexley et. al. *Arms to fights, arms to protect. Women speak out about conflict.* London: Panos. 1995.
18. These are the words of the Pierre Sané, the Secretary General of Amnesty International, at the workshop Conflict, Development and Ethnicity during the NGO-meeting at the Global Coalition For Africa. 25 November 1995.
19. Arcel, Libby Tata et. al, *Psyco-social help to war-victims: women refugees and their families.* Copenhagen: IRTC. 1995. pp. 13-14.

2. THE WAR, THE SCHOOL AND REFUGEE CHILDREN'S MENTAL HEALTH PROTECTION

Anica Mikus Kos

Introduction

In spring 1992 Slovenia registered about 70.000 refugees from Bosnia and Herzegovina and it was estimated that there were about additional 30.000 not registered. In autumn 1992 the primary school for refugee children started to function and about 9.000 children aged 7 to 15 attended 'Refugee schools', which have been a system parallel to the regular Slovene elementary school system. The Slovene Ministry of Education was the umbrella organization and the legal responsible institution for refugee schools. At this ministry a counsellor from Sarajevo has worked together with the Slovene counsellor on the system of refugee schools. The teachers have been refugees themselves. Among 450 teachers about 50% were professional educators, others were engineers, lawyers, physicians or members of other professions or students. They started to work as volunteers, later they have received minimal fees.

The Mental Health Team of the Counselling Centre for Children, Adolescents and Parents in Ljubljana started to provide mental health help to refugee children and adolescents from their arrival to Slovenia in spring 1992 on.

The work of the Mental Health Team was run with the agreement of the Ministry of Education of the Republic Slovenia and coordinated with the Ministry. The Mental Health Team was composed of pedagogues, special teachers, psychologists and child psychiatrists.

The basic question then was how to provide mental health help to ten thousands of children being all scared, stressed, experiencing important losses and many of them being deeply traumatized. Taking into consideration the figures and the mental health condition of refugee children it was clear that the existing Slovene mental health services would not be able to treat this population. On the other side, it soon became evident that refugees were not prone to seek mental health help in the existing institutions. Therefore new models had to be elaborated, models of population oriented and outreaching mental health activities.

The Mental Health Team developed some of those models. In the first year the most important and efficient were:

1. Mobile mental health teams visiting collective shelters for refugees and providing different mental health activities with preventive, protective and therapeutic contents.
2. Mental health activities in schools.

These two models permitted the access of at least some mental health help to the majority of refugee children and to many parents. This paper presents the description of the functioning and of the role of the primary school for refugee children in Slovenia and the model and effects of the collaboration of the Mental Health Team with the primary schools. The message which our team wants to transmit to those who can do something for the protection of the well-being of refugee children and for their mental health protection is that the organization of elementary school has the highest priority within the care for refugees and that introducing psychosocial activities in schools is the best if not the only way to ensure some mental health protection of a great number of stressed children and children at risk.

The social and psychological function of the refugee school

The scope of the school in refugee situations is far wider and more significant than that of a school under normal conditions. The school is not just a provider of knowledge and a facility the children have for not losing another school year. In the case of refugees from Bosnia and Herzegovina, we can state that it was the framework structuring the entire life of the children and the entire refugee community in Slovenia.
The school is the organization which has made lives of refugee children more normal. It is the only institutional structure that has remained from refugees' pre-war life. The complete break with the normal life is bound to have a severe psychological impact on children. The regularly run school narrowed the gap between the normal life and life in exile. It proved to be of great importance for children's psychological condition.

School fills daily children's and teachers' life with activity, it gives structure and meaning to each day. Inactivity is one of the greatest hardships of refugee life. People have been pushed into a state of idleness and inactivity by external circumstances. They do not go out to work. There are no normal household activities. There is no cooking, working outdoors in the garden or in the fields. There are no jobs. The refugees' inactivity is also psychologically conditioned: it is a result of hopelessness, complete dependence on others, depression. Idleness, time wasting and emptiness enhance passivity and deepen the state of depression. Every meaningful, organized, regular activity, therefore, represents an important protective psychosocial factor.

The school is a life environment differing from that of the refugee collective shelters or host family environment. It is a place where the child does not only listen to the stories about disasters that have hit or may hit family members or friends, where he does not just watch war scenes on television, does not only listen to the worried adults talking about war events. The school has a different content. A child's thoughts are engaged in the pursuit of other topics, his intellectual and experiential world is getting broader and filled with new ideas. The school broadens his horizons and thought, which would otherwise remain restricted to the war events and the narrow world of the collective shelter or host family environment.

School directs children's thoughts to the future, to the next lesson for which they need to do some home-work, to the end of the school year.

School facilitates encounters with new, often interesting and attractive, people. One can make new friends, find new company so that the circle of social contacts gets broader and more diverse. The people one meets are no longer just family members, the extended family or people with whom you are sharing whatever accommodation you have.

School means acquiring new knowledge and insights, developing new interests. School makes the child mentally and emotionally active, awakens his curiosity and motivates him for further intellectual and social development.

School helps the child to develop his working habits. In normal life most children would have some household duties to do, but not in refugee life. School brings into the idleness of refugee life the changing rhythm of work and rest.

Attending school, having the status of a pupil with defined obligations counteracts the feeling of total dependence and helplessness. The pupil is, to a certain degree, gaining control over his life. He is at least partly relieved of dependence on others. It greatly depends on himself whether he will or will not do his homework or learn the lesson, what mark he will get, whether he will pass the class or not.

School tends to stabilize life. In the unpredictable situation in which it is impossible to know what the next day will bring, what the fate of the family, village or community will be, what will happen on the war and political scene - the stabilizing elements, those bringing predictability, are of utmost significance for the psychological condition of both children and adults. The refugee children, characteristically, lack the feeling of security, which can be in part explained by the unexpectedness of the terrible events and shocks they have experienced, but partly also by the uncertainty of their present life situation. It is not clear when the war will finish, whether father and grandmother who remained in Bosnia are still alive, where the family will live in the future. School with its regular rhythm and predictability enhances the feeling of safety in children.

When one is a refugee, one's self-esteem is likely to suffer. Both children and adults experience injustice and humiliation, they are deprived of their material and social attributes which support one's positive self-image. At school children partly recuperate their social role, their rights as students and they receive recognition for their work. The school which makes it possible for a child to be successful in a certain subject or in an extra-curricular activity, the teacher who likes and respects the child, can considerably raise the child's self-esteem.

The school for refugee children from Bosnia and Herzegovina with the teachers from their native country give the children the feeling of belonging to a social structure, which constitutes part of a broader domestic culture and social structure, that of one's home country. It enhances in children cultural awareness and the sense of belonging to their community.

At school a child meets many people who may help him with his developmental and psychological problems. These are first of all his teachers and schoolmates.

The school acts as a remedial agent for all refugee children, but it is also a rich source of psychological help for children with serious emotional problems, especially for those whose parents are - for whatever reason - unable to provide the needed support and consolation.A male teacher was especially important to children without fathers; he may occasionally assume the role of father.

Many primary school refugee children are suffering from severe traumas and have deep emotional problems and the school is the place where these children can easily be discovered. Psychological problems of many children might have gone unnoticed, had the children not been attending school. All children have been included in schools - children living in collective shelters and those living in host families family, those with the status of refugee and those without it. Therefore the school was a good place for detecting children who were seriously traumatized and children with other serious psychological disorders. Teachers were good diagnostician and they detected many children with emotional and learning disorders. Teachers come across all children who need help. The teachers, who are with children for several hours every day, are, thus, able to help the children.

Some parents do not see the suffering of their children. Others do, but because of their own grief and despair they may lack the energy to help their children. Some parents do not know how to help their children. Practically, in the first months of asylum life the school was the only social space where some help could be provided and the teachers were the only available helpers outside the family.

The teachers are in touch with parents and can exert beneficial influence on the relationship between the parents and the children even those who are not going to school. They could counsel parents about the upbringing of their children.

Soon after the start of the school, the important normalizing, corrective, and social therapeutic role of the refugee school became evident. We consider that in the first year of war these functions of the school were more important than the educational ones. The school represented an island of regularity and predictability in the totally uncertain situation of the refugee population, an important element of normalization and a considerable resource of psychosocial and psychological support for children, parents and teachers.

The emotional reactions of refugee children

The children who have experienced war and emigration often show symptoms of emotional disorders. The most frequent symptoms are: fear, sadness, sleep disorders, various psychosomatic complaints, restlessness, irritability, aggressive behaviour, regressive behaviour, apathy, lack of interest, mistrust, lack of self-confidence, memory problems, impaired concentration, other learning difficulties.

All these phenomena were present in refugee children when they arrived to Slovenia. But a remarkable decline in difficulties appeared some weeks after the start of the school. Concerning the frequency, the intensity and the duration of common symptoms of psychological distress and adaptation disorders our expectations had been much more pessimist than the reality proved to be. We expected the children to have serious school adaptation problems at the start. As the children had not been to school for months, we believed many would have difficulty getting used to the school discipline once again and meeting school requirements. We thought, it would take quite a while for them to redevelop working habits. It is true that at the beginning there were more problems with refugee children than in ordinary schools but these problems were not beyond the teachers' control. The main problems were increased restlessness and concentration and memory problems. But the situation was considerably better then we expected. The remedial effects of the school were much more important than the adaptation difficulties. After only a few weeks it became evident that the school had a most soothing effect on children. Their behaviour had improved, their learning abilities were raised.

Fear of school and non-attendance appeared occasionally. Sometimes it had the feature of school phobia. Many refugee children have experienced a lot of fear because of the war, they have suffered the loss of a member of the family or uncertainty about the fate of their fathers or brothers, so there is no wonder they were afraid of leaving their mothers when going to school, especially if the school was far away. The child's non-attendance of lessons was sometimes caused by the fear of the mother or some other adult in charge of the child who - again under the influence of the present and past horrors - was afraid that something might happen to the child on the way to school or at school. Besides, some parents did not want to be separated from the children because they felt more secure if the children were with them.

Even under normal circumstances many children have learning problems or lack of motivation for learning. The children who have experienced traumatic events, who chronically live under stress, who have spent a lot of emotional and mental energy for adjustment to life in Slovenia, who have no quiet place of their own to learn, who have not been to school for a long time, certainly could be expected to have learning difficulties. In many children from Bosnia and Herzegovina learning difficulties manifested themselves in concentration and memory disorders. They were most common in the first months of school. The teachers reported that some children could not remember the name of their school or teacher from Bosnia and Herzegovina, that their capacity of memorizing the school subjects was poor. Severely traumatized children and adolescents whose fathers were missed specially complained about incapacity to concentrate. Some children had specific learning problems, most common of which were dyslexia and dysgraphia. Some parents would enrol children who had previously attended a special school for mentally retarded children without informing the teachers. But in general, pupils accomplished their work satisfactorily.

How the children felt about the school is obvious from their statements. At the beginning they regretted working with a reduced curriculum, not having gymnastics or some other subjects. Many children complained about not having their own books. Some were depressed by the unpleasant physical conditions of work (dirt, noise). It should be said that many schools were established in improvised class rooms in defective military barracks. Some complained about the differences between the treatment of the Slovene children and the children from Bosnia In cases where their lessons were held on the premises of the Slovene school; they would say, for example: "They are getting a meal at school, but we are not". Still, the children were aware of what was good and useful in the school. When asked what they liked best about the school, they would name their teacher, the pleasure of going to school, satisfaction at not having to always be present at the discussions about the war, the joy of having the company of other children. In other words, the benefits of the school which we presented as protective factors were seen as such by the children themselves.

What we did and how we worked

The initial premise of the mental health team was that the primary school embracing all refugee children aged from 7-15 was the most reliable structure for the provision of mental health support to an enormous number of children. Transmitting knowledge, energy and time of mental health workers to teachers and motivating them for the role of psychosocial helper was presumed to be the most economic and efficient investment of a few of us in refugee children's mental health protection. Therefore we developed a model of continuous and intense work with teachers. The aims of this work were:

a. To educate and sensitize teachers to recognize emotional and learning problems in children.
b. To give them some practical knowledge how to help children with emotional, behavioral and learning problems.
c. To instruct them about crisis situations and intense traumas and the possibilities of help.
d. To provide personal psychological support for teachers who were themselves under chronic stress of the refugee situation and many of them experiencing personal losses like violent death of a member of the family.
e. To provide direct professional mental health help to children with special needs, psychosocial problems and learning difficulties (at least to some of them).
f. To reach at least a part of parents (on meetings for parents, in individual contacts).
g. To improve teachers' educational capacities and skills.

Our programme comprised of working with teachers (e.g. workshops, seminars, counselling for their professional problems and for their personal problems, support), working with children (e.g. diagnostic, counselling, individual and group therapeutic work, herbal medicine, providing facilities for physical activities, cultural activities, other occupation), and working with parents (e.g. meetings of parents in schools, information, counselling). Our goal was to reach all teachers teaching in the schools for the children from Bosnia and Herzegovina in Slovenia and, thus, indirectly all refugee children attending primary schools and their parents.

As soon as the school started we began visiting schools all over Slovenia; there were 52 schools. We held courses and workshops for teachers. Alongside with courses and workshops, we started having talks with parents at parents' meetings. The teachers wanted to have consultations for individual children and examinations of the children who had learning difficulties and behaviour problems, those who were too restless or displayed apathy or grief. In the work with the teachers we found out that they needed help in two areas: in the field of psychological knowledge and in the field of pedagogical knowledge. They lacked pedagogical knowledge since about 50% of the teachers had not received any pedagogical training. As the school year went on, teachers required more knowledge in education, which we considered as a good sign. So we added to workshops and seminars with psychological contents some ones with educational contents. But the most important source of educational knowledge for non-teachers were their teachers colleagues. Most of the training of new teachers was done by the teachers themselves. Teachers would help the 'non-teacher' to prepare for their lessons.A lot of effort went into learning of the new profession on the part of the 'new' teachers.

The teaching situation differed a great deal from a normal school situation. The psychological, professional, organizational, material conditions were out of comparison with the normal educational conditions. It demanded a much higher degree of creativeness from the teacher. But the teachers showed unbelievable good will, energy and inventiveness to overcome difficulties. The members of the Mental health team were eager to give the merited recognition to teachers and to enhance their motivation.

Similarly, in the domain of psychology, I was surprised by the sensitivity of the teachers faced with the emotional problems of the children, how well they understood them and how willing most of them were to help children. Nevertheless, we persisted with the psychological education of the teachers believing that by relating some specific knowledge we could perhaps contribute to their human wisdom and their innate ability to help the fellow human being in distress.

The teachers received some specific instructions for their work related to the war situation and to the circumstances of the refugee life. If, for example, the teacher learned that something tragic happened to the child, e.g. that his father was killed, he should try to help the child by talking to him warmly, undertaking common activities or with body contacts. In a critical situation human attention and understanding help. It helps if the teacher gets in touch with the child's mother or some other member of the family in order to discuss with them how to make it easier for the child to bear the trauma.

A frequent question was whether it was necessary that every single child who has had a bad experience or suffered a tragic loss should talk about them? By repeated processing of the traumatic event through narration, games or drawings remedial effects can be achieved. The prerequisite, however, is that the helper is a warm person with the ability to understand the child's psychological difficulties, a person able to express his empathy in a manner the child understands. The conversation should be carried out by a teacher who has a good relationship with the child and is strong enough to be with the child who had experienced something very sad. For the processing of the traumatic event to be beneficial, it is essential that the child feels secure. An important thing to remember is that the conversation with the child should end in a soothing way, giving the child's thoughts and feelings a positive and optimistic direction. It is possible, for example, to point out what is positive in the child's life, how to overcome sadness and anxiety, to give him practical guidelines, to help the child to face actively his psychological problems. There are, however, children who simply do not want to talk about their experiences. Some of them seem to be able to cope with their traumas on their own. Such children should not be forced to talk, they should only know they have a possibility to talk if they felt like it.

Some children have the habit of telling their story over and over again, which may irritate other children and bring about intolerant and aggressive reactions, which in turn will make the compulsive speaker feel even more lonely and misunderstood. To help him, the child should be stopped from repeating the story to his peers. He should be listened to by the teacher who can understand the child's need to talk.

The children need to be given the opportunity to speak about their school in Bosnia an Herzegovina, about their village, about their town, about their home, about how they lived at home, to compare life in their country with life in Slovenia, the previous school with the present.

The lessons should include topics related to the country in which the children are living, about its culture and customs. This makes it easier for the children to adapt to the new environment and to overcome embarrassment in front of the natives of the country which has given them shelter. Connections with the Slovene schools and with the Slovene children whenever possible will contribute considerably to the adaptation and the feeling of security in the asylum country.

During the lessons the teacher should not use texts dealing with the war as they evoke intense emotions. Texts which provoke feelings of adversity grounded on

nationality should be omitted. When discussing war and the fate of refugees the teacher should point out the optimistic perspectives, examples of humanity and help the child see the positive happenings.
The teacher should be sensitive to national, religious and other tensions which may appear in the classroom. The basic values propagated should be peace and tolerance. Generalizations, such as 'all members of a certain nation are bad people' must not be made. It is important to stress humanity and show how it comes to expression in the war and refugee situations. The teacher has a lot of possibilities for moral education, education for peace and tolerance among different nations, different cultures and different philosophies of life. In cases when intolerance or hate appeared (which was rare), the unfairness and danger of generalizations were discussed. For instance: "Is it true that all Serbs are evil? Let us think about your school mates in the village you lived in Bosnia. Name them and describe them". In this exercise it became evident that there were kind children and good mates among Serbian children as well. It is important to educate children in the spirit of solidarity and make them assume the role of helpers of people in their community - the old, the sick and the young.

It is necessary to mobilize help of as many refugees as possible - parents, other adults, young people - all those who are able to help the school in its running.
If the teachers themselves have serious personal and professional problems, they should look for help. This will be beneficial for themselves as well as for their pupils.

We wanted to prevent bad pupils from suffering additional traumas on account of their school failure. Some teachers became rather demanding, which was, on the whole, good for the children. Sometimes, however, this resulted in too strict an evaluation of a child's work and too much pressure on the child. It also happened that children with poor school performance came under a lot of pressure on the part of their parents, who would resort to punishment. I remember a mother saying: "I beat him to make him learn. And at the same time I feel sorry for him. I beat him and shed tears at the same time." Our message to both the teacher and the parents was, in such cases: Your children have suffered a lot, do not make them unhappy by punishing them for school failure. Think of how you could help them instead.

Towards the end of the year we paid special attention to the children with learning difficulties. Psychologists and special teachers examined the children in some schools and, on the basis of their findings, discussed with the teachers what to do in a particular case; should they organize special help, prolong lessons over the summer period or make the child repeat the grade. The possibility to consult somebody made it easier for teachers to take a decision. It was not easy to say to the child who lost his father or to the child's mother that the child will not be able to go to the next grade. Therefore, the psychologist's and special teacher's opinion occasionally meant moral support for the teacher.
Sometimes the mental health team helped the school with some intervention which affected the functioning of the school, for instance the substitution of an inadequate teacher. Some unforseen components became part of our activities, as providing individual material help to children with special needs. Such as buying colours for a depressed child who is a gifted painter, helping parents of a child with cancer to buy special food for the child, buying some sport requisites, giving money for travel fees for a lady teacher who visited her wounded husband in the hospital in Croatia.

Teachers' mental health activities

Through psychological education we also wanted to give the teachers something useful for themselves - for better coping and overcoming proper psychological traumas. The most important teachers' psychosocial tasks were:

1. To create in the class an atmosphere of comfort, trust, friendship.
2. To prevent new school related stressful situations (fear, humiliation because of learning difficulties).
3. To teaching children to seek and accept help from others.
4. To help children with learning problems to improve their school work, their attitude to learning and schooling and their self esteem.
5. To pay special attention to children with difficulties in peer relationships: to help them to improve their social skills, to teach them appropriate behaviour and to promote more accepting and supportive attitudes towards these children in the peer group; social games were favourite techniques.
6. To motivate children to express their feelings and to discuss in an open way problems linked to the refugee situation, to losses and other stresses. In such

discussions positive aspects of children's life in asylum and positive perspectives had to be exposed and underlined. Children were motivated to discover themselves such positive elements. This was difficult for some teachers who were themselves deeply depressed. It became difficult for the majority of teachers in periods when hope for the end of the war and for return vanished after being raised by some political contracts. In such situations some teacher asked the counsellors: "What should we tell them?"

7. To support children who experienced heavy losses like the death of a parent or sibling. The support was mainly manifested by sympathy, more verbal and nonverbal contacts, more time spend together, efforts to activate the child for sport, artistic or other activities.
8. To refer children and family members to mental health professionals when needed - to psychologists, psychiatrists, special teachers who visited collective shelters and refugee schools as members of mobile mental health teams.

It was not easy for the teachers either

As mentioned before, nearly all teachers working in the refugee school were refugees themselves afflicted by war experience and hardships of refugee life. They also lost their property, their social position, members of the family. At several international conferences we could hear the opinion that a traumatized person is not able to help others. When I was telling international audiences about the school for refugee children, several experts maintained that without receiving psychotherapy the refugee teachers are not able to help children. But in reality this was not the case. The vast majority of the teachers from Bosnia and Herzegovina have done their professional and humane tasks to the full benefit of the children, even though they had received no psychotherapy, which - needless to say, they had no possibility of obtaining. The majority of them would even not consent to psychotherapy at least before their became more familiar with the members and the activities of the Mental Health team. As other refugees, they answered to the offer of psychotherapeutic help by saying that they were not crazy, they just normally responded to a crazy and totally abnormal situation.

Teachers had a manyfold hard time. They were working under the burden of their own sad destiny and under the burden of numerous tragic fates of their pupils, their pupils' and their families' losses, their grief and traumas becoming often teachers' own inner preoccupations. Some situations were particularly difficult for teachers. For example: In many Muslim families the death of the father was concealed to the child. Everybody in the collective shelter and all teachers knew that the child's father was killed, but the child was not told about it. Teachers often asked what to do, because they had the feeling that the child knows about her or his father death, but had nobody to speak with about her or his grief.

The psychological affliction of teachers was further aggravated by their present life and work situations. They were living and working under unfavourable conditions. Teaching often had to be done without the necessary teaching Aids. There were not enough books, notebooks, when the school started sometimes there was not even enough chalk. For their work the teachers received very little payment, there would be several months when they received none at all.

As many teachers had not any pedagogical training, they had to learn a lot and work hard in order to prepare their lessons.

In some collective shelters the teachers were sharing accommodation with their pupils, in others they were not exempted from the duty of cleaning common rooms although they contributed to the community no doubt so much more than they would by just cleaning corridors and toilets.

Teachers had a number of problems with parents. They were disappointed by the fact that some parents, especially at the beginning, failed to enrol their children in school or make them attend lessons regularly, that parents were not interested in their school progress. Some of the parents' reactions, conditioned by refugee life, were especially painful. The teachers, who were actually working as volunteers and were sacrificing a lot of their time for their lessons understandably felt hurt when some parents were unwilling to give them or the school any help. It happened, for example, that a mother refused to look after a teacher's child for the time she was teaching or that parents refused to help arrange and clean schoolrooms.

Among the staff of some schools there were also conflicts, which had various causes. Sometimes the conflicts arose between the teachers and non-teachers, sometimes they had to do with the nationality issue, the question which alphabet and which language ought to be taught. Occasionally the conflicts reflected rivalry among teachers or other problems that appear in normal life conditions, which we considered as a good sign of normalization of the psychosocial situation. But the mental health team offered help in conflict resolution when conflict aggravated and threatened to have a destructive effects. As we were aware of the great importance of the school, but also how fragile and vulnerable its structure was, we did our best to help to resolve such conflicts. If several teachers had stopped working because of the conflicts, this might have meant the end of the school in a collective shelter or area, which would seriously afflict hundreds of children.

What helped teachers to survive

When we analyzed together with teachers what could be of help to them for overcoming their difficulties, the following protective processes were identified. Mutual help among colleagues, family members and friends represents the main source of energy needed to overcome despair and apathy. It helps to be able to talk to someone who is stronger, stronger perhaps only at a given moment.
Among most important identified positive factors was the moral and emotional satisfaction the teachers obtained from their work. On the courses they attended they would often say: "I don't know how I would manage without doing in this work."
Positive feedback on the part of participants in the educational process (the children and parents) provides a further motivation and can counterbalance the unfavourable conditions of work and bad experiences. A collective evaluation of the quality and effects of teachers' work helps at moments of apathy. A recurrent personal reflection of one's own work and of the significance of the refugee school may prevent teachers from having a dangerously pessimist picture of the happening. An important cause of satisfaction in teachers was the awareness of the positive impact of their work on children and the whole refugee community. The functions of the teachers in the refugee schools were much broader, complex and important than in ordinary life. They acted as psychologists, social workers and substitute parents. Teachers often told us with satisfaction and pride how attached the children became to them, how small children longed for physical contacts, would want to hold their hands etc. In many such cases it was the teacher who was able to comfort and console the child. In some cases the teacher became councillor, to whom parents would turn for advice on educational problems, personal problems, when not knowing what to say to an unhappy child, how to console him or bring the news about death of a parent. Many school

directors took over the responsibility for medical care and other out-of-school matters to do with their pupils. They often had contacts with the humanitarian and voluntary organizations and individual volunteers. The school structure served as a basis for different types of help to the refugee community.
Personal development and acquisition of new pedagogical, psychological and other knowledge contributed to overcoming the feelings of depression and exhaustion.
It must be said here, that in the refugee situation the teachers were the only people who have preserved their professional social roles. None of the other refugees could take on any employment. Those who worked illegally, had to do jobs that were beneath their level of qualification. The teachers, on the other hand, remained teachers or persons from other professions became teachers. They were the only segment of adults among the refugees who had regular working obligations and attributes pertaining to the professional social role.

Supporting teachers

One of the most important objective of the project was supporting teachers in their educational professional role and in their role of psychosocial helpers. It is difficult to describe the atmosphere of hopelessness and despair in the collective shelters and in the economically deprived refugee families living outside shelters in overcrowded flats. Refugees usually live outside collective shelters with members of family who had migrated to Slovenia before the war to undertake an unqualified work. So they were in a very poor economic situation when the members of extended family arrived as refugees to invade their small flat. Teachers were influenced by such conditions as well. To the general stresses of the war and refugee situation, specific difficulties connected with teachers' function were added.
The Mental Health Team tried to provide psychosocial support to teachers, to encourage them and rise their optimism, self-esteem and sense of dignity. Maybe by involving them in mental health activities we helped them in these directions. The trust of the mental health professionals concerning teachers' capacities to perform the new role properly and partnership in collaboration with Slovene mental health workers were certainly rewarding and gratifying for teachers.

The second approach consisted in enhancing their coping capacities and personal growth by providing knowledge, insights, cognitive changes, coping techniques. Attending workshops and seminars in a normal and comfortable environment of some cheap hotel or summer resort and being treated respectfully by Slovene mental health workers, contributed to their well-being. One teacher expressed it by saying: "This is the first time since I have been a refugee that I have felt as a respected human being with my own dignity.". And they often repeated that workshops and seminars refilled their batteries for the next two months.

The seminars and workshops were also a good opportunity for exchange of views and experience between the teachers working in various collective shelters and schools, as specially as refugees were not supposed to leave collective shelters in the first year of asylum. The second practical limitation was the lack of funds which made it impossible for the teachers to make trips around Slovenia.
Supporting financially, practically and morally the realization on some of teachers' incentives for different psychosocial activities of the school was an important means of motivation.

Evaluation of the project and final thoughts

It was really admirable that in the first year of the totally improvised refugee school so many teachers managed to do an excellent job, which required a lot of personal sacrifice and goodwill. We could say that the first year of the refugee school or as we use to say in a familiar way of 'Bosnian school' was inspired by teachers' altruism and enthusiasm. The motivation of teachers was certainly also nurtured from their social position - they were the only persons effecting a normal regular and established social and professional role. They were also aware of the importance of the school for children and they certainly received a lot of satisfaction and gratification from their work.
We consider that the social and psychosocial function of the school for refugee children from Bosnia and Herzegovina in Slovenia proved the theoretical findings about the protective role of the school in children facing chronic adversities.

But the second school-year starting in September 1993 soon showed signs of deterioration of the refugee school system. The situation in schools was the reflection of the global war and refugee situation. More and more people lost their hope to return to Bosnia, they became more and more passive and depressed. Many people left Slovenia for other Western European countries, Canada or other countries. Those who left were the most educated, the most energetic and those who stayed in Slovenia were mostly helpless people, from rural areas of Bosnia and Herzegovina. A great number of teachers left as well. The danger that the organizational structure will fall apart was present. Besides teachers were not paid for their work and many of them were without any income. Many other people succeeded to get some illegal work which was the source of at least some minimum earning of money. Teachers could not engage in such activities because they had to work in schools. Towards the end of the school-year 1993/94 some foreign money arrived, so very modest fees could be given to teachers. But then many good teachers had already left Slovenia. In the second year of the refugee primary school the activities of the Mental Health Team were even intensified, because the school was so much endangered. But we often felt that the impact of our efforts to counterpoint the destructive social and psychosocial forces deteriorating the school, was very limited.

This departure of a certain number of teachers was a source of frustration for all participants of the project - children, remaining teachers and counsellors. This loss has been many fold - emotional, moral and substantial in terms of taking away the acquired knowledge, and reducing the impact of the total amount of teachers' knowledge. New teachers took the places of the old ones and we continued to work with them.

One of the premises of the project was also that teachers will take their knowledge to Bosnia and Herzegovina where it will be urgently needed. But obviously many teachers will never return to their native land.

The presented project of introducing mental health activities in refugee schools is not a research project and therefore a scientific evaluation can not be expected. But even if it were a scientific project, a fair evaluation of its effects would be very difficult. In the tragic natural experiment which refugees from Bosnia and Herzegovina are facing, there are so many influences which determine the state of heart and mind of people, that it is impossible to evaluate reliably the impact of one intervention.

The project could be understood as an action research project. Our evaluation is mainly based on discussions with teachers and our observations of their behaviour and of children's behaviour. Our impression and estimation is that the mental health project had an important impact on the functioning of teachers and schools. One effect was that nearly all teachers (about 420 of them) knew the members of the Mental Health Team and addressed themselves to mental health workers when they needed any form of help. Another positive sign was that practically all teachers attended workshops, and they pushed us to organize new workshops.

The question remains whether teachers detected emotional wounds in the majority of children. As the Mental Health Team has been preoccupied with helping activities we have not run epidemiologic screening. This question is relevant not only because of epidemiologic researches demonstrate that the population of children identified by the teachers is only a part of the whole population of children having emotional and psychosocial disorders. There is an even more important additional aspect: the characteristic emotional answer of a considerable number of refugee children from Bosnia and Herzegovina is what refugee teachers name 'hidden sorrow'. Many children bearing sadness do not demonstrate usual symptoms of emotional disorders, they play and function normally, but in there written texts they express sorrow and longing for their native land, they often cry when they hear Bosnian songs or when they talk about their family members and homes in the native land. We can admit that many of those children were not referred to mental health workers, but they did profit from the general mental health attitude of the school.

The refugee school can also be regarded as an interesting experiment, from which both pedagogy and psychology could learn a lot. It is a pity we do not have sufficient time, will and energy to try and answer questions like: 'How much can children learn under conditions which greatly differ from ordinary schools - in a considerably shorter time, with a considerably smaller number of lessons, with teachers who are not pedagogues by profession, without normal educational facilities and Aids? How is it possible that refugee children have functioned so well at school in spite of the tragic events they had witnessed, in spite of grief, losses, emotional traumas and adverse living conditions in exile and adaptation requirements? And many others.

3. VIOLENCE AGAINST WOMEN

Annemiek J.M. Richters[1]

Introduction

The problem of women and violence is not only a health, but also a human rights and a development issue. Human rights and development in general have increasingly come to be seen as complementary concerns and mutually reinforcing practices. In fact, 'human rights' together with 'democracy', 'good governance', 'peoples' rights' and 'sustainability' have become the new catchwords of development cooperation between the North and the South. I shall discuss what type of linkages between human rights and development are most favourable for the protection of women's human rights, particularly women's right to freedom from gender violence. Gender violence being defined as violence directed against women or which affects women disproportionably *because* they are women.

Gender violence, being a complex issue, calls for a comprehensive response. The importance of being selective, however, must also be underlined. What appears critical in constructing a strategic plan for combatting gender violence is having a comprehensive view of what is required to be effective, together with an appreciation of the contextual possibilities and limitations. An ineffective design of the strategy chosen to tackle gender violence in a particular context can stem from focusing either too narrowly or too broadly on the problem[2].

The complexity of gender violence is addressed by shedding some light on the intricate linkages between gender violence as a development, a human rights and a health issue, approached each time from a different angle. A selection of general recommendations is also made. They are only given, however, as guidelines for determining what is most needed in a particular socio-cultural context. The therapeutic guidelines developed in the West for working with trauma survivors, for instance, may not be applicable in non-Western cultures. More research in this area is a sine qua non for development agencies who choose to make a contribution to the rebuilding of individual lives and communities shattered by violence in such a way that at least some of the many cycles of conflict and violence in the present world may eventually be broken.

The right to development

The 'right to development' was introduced by the Banjul Charter as one of the elements of a so-called 'third generation' of human rights, the other elements being the right to peace, to a clean environment and to sharing the common heritage of mankind.

The watchword of the first generation of human rights was *liberty*, notably liberty from governmental intrusions on individuals; of the second generation it was *equality*, for which governments were to pursue collective achievement of betterment. Third generation rights, by contrast, involve *solidarity*, both between Southern States as a group, and between all states in general. Where the first and second generation of human rights are dependent on the organization of separate nation states and, as far as their socio-economic rights are concerned, partly also on their economic development, international cooperation is a first requirement for the third generation of human rights.

For proponents of human rights in Africa and Asia - and most particularly African and Asian governments - the three generations of human rights are interdependent. The connections are tenuous, however. In practice, the three sorts of rights are rather competing than complementary. The first and second generation of human rights are easily engulfed by the concern for development. There is a reluctance to relinquish some incremental economic growth in favour of more immediate satisfaction of human rights. Increasing the goods and services available to governments in the South or within Southern economies will increase the enjoyment of social human rights only if these resources are equitably distributed. In developing countries, the concern for social, economic and cultural rights in its turn often engulfs the right to liberty. Many governments are prepared to deny certain civil and political rights in their own countries in the desire to enhance economic growth and national unity. The World Bank and the International Monetary Fund (IMF) have, indirectly, encouraged military and one-party dictatorships. Opposition to the World Bank and IMF programs by farmers and workers has been brutally suppressed[3].

Thus, rather than marking 'the penetration of human rights into the field of development', as it is often presented, the right to development in fact represents the engulfing of human rights by the concerns of development - that is, economic development; human rights are transformed into just another political and ideological instrument for seeking progress in the New International Economic Order. This kind of progress has brought with it the destruction of nature, the destruction of ways of life and the degradation of women. If the right to development is to be promoted, new criteria and measurements should accompany this effort[4]. This amounts to finding the *proper* way to link human rights and development. Donnelly[5] argues that we would do better to shift our attention away from the right to development and towards the topic of incorporating human rights concerns into the difficult task of national development planning. The right to development conflates rights and development, rather than suggesting strategies for integrating these two related, but quite distinct, concerns.

Development for women is development for society

It is now recognized by men and women alike that women are a major force for change[6]. Development strategies which limit the ability of women to achieve their real potential are also strategies which limit the potential of communities and nations. This is well expressed by the male writer and film maker Sembène Ousmane from Senegal:

> " Without the liberation of women, Africa will never be free. Real revolution is impossible without women. Nothing is more revolutionary than strong feelings of love. We are driven into a corner by religion. Every religion suffocates women in their development, just as every regime censures artists. As long as the African woman is not really free, while forced marriages still exist, and the master-servant relationship is found, there will be no question of any change. (...) That we still survive is thanks to the women in the villages. They are the backbone of the country. If they don't take action, we shall all perish. Men will never change, unless women want us to. Men have the power, they fought for it. Why should they share it then? That is what women should fight for"[7].

There are, however, many constraints to women's full participation in society and their fight for a change in the way societies are developing. One of them is the problem of gender violence. The United Nations (UN) began to recognize this problem within the context of the UN Decade for Women. This particular international concern culminated in the Nairobi Forward Looking Strategies for the Advancement of Women: equality - development - peace (FLS), which acknowledged the responsibility of governments and all members of society to eradicate violence.

The FLS document, adopted by consensus at the final conference of the UN Decade for Women, held in Nairobi in 1985, remains the strongest UN document on violence against women in relation to development goals. It includes paragraph 258 which calls for the creation of preventive policies and institutionalized means of assistance to women who fall victim to the various forms of violence perceived in everyday life in all cultures. This resolution acknowledges that "women are beaten, mutilated, burned, sexually abused, and raped" and that such violence is "a major obstacle to the achievement of the objectives of the Decade and should be given special attention".

In the FLS, the concept of peace is defined both as absence of war and direct violence, and as absence of structural violence. The FLS thus adopts the concept of positive peace instead of negative peace. It is stated that sustainable peace cannot be achieved without eliminating violence at all levels, including violence against women. The Nairobi FLS paper is the first unanimously adopted intergovernmental document in which the concept of violence is defined in a comprehensive way, and where the links between the use of violence at personal and international levels are recognized. In paragraph 257 it states: "The questions of women and peace and the meaning of peace for women cannot be separated from the broader question of relationships between women and men in all spheres of life and family." Increasingly, women are realizing that in order to change society, they must begin within the family and the community. "Women's capacity to challenge the men in their families, their communities, or their political movements will be a key to remaking the world"[8].

Gender violence as an obstacle to development

In addition to causing untold human misery and affecting women's human rights, violence is often a direct obstacle to women's participation in development projects. Women cannot fully devote their labour or creative ideas to development when they are burdened with the physical and psychological scars of violence. During the Global Tribunal on Violations of Women's Human Rights (Vienna, June 1993) Bernice See of the Philippines spoke of the often-ignored economic impact of gender-based violence, asking, "How many opportunities have been lost because a woman could not physically, emotionally or mentally afford to go to work? How much is our productivity affected because we have to take time out to heal?"[9] Violence drains women's energies, and may undermine all women's efforts to further their own, and their community's, development. Development does not occur where domestic violence keeps a woman from participating in development projects, where violence outside and inside the home threatens and prevents freedom of movement, assembly and political participation, where force is used to deprive her of earnings, or fear of sexual assault prevents her from taking a job or attending a public function.

Even though it is obvious that gender violence is indeed an obstacle to development for women, case studies to illustrate this are still hard to find in the literature. Gender violence in development projects has apparently been a blind spot. The available case studies are all of very recent date. The Center for Women's Global Leadership[10], gives as an example that a revolving loan project of the Working Women's Forum in Madras almost collapsed when its most energetic participants dropped out after being beaten by their husbands. The men saw the women's growing empowerment as a threat to their control. Faced with the same problem, the Association for the Development and Integration of Women in Lima succeeded in its work by initiating programmes that combine income-generating schemes with legal aid to battered wives and women abandoned by their partners[11]. Pronk[12] refers to a report by Mathangani from Kenya who writes: "We have instances when the husband burns the wife's hands if she is a tailor, so that she no longer can earn her living"[13].

To be able to give and take their full share in development projects, women must first overcome the violence against them. The problem is, however, that violence keeps women economically dependent and exploited, while economic dependence and exploitation render them unable to combat violence. The relationship is apparently circular, and it takes a great deal of energy, intelligence and risk-taking on the part of victimized women to break this circle. Women's development organizations such as Match International[14] have made it their policy to support women's efforts worldwide to end violence against women and thus help to create the conditions necessary for development and social justice for all humanity. Like other 'women in development' policies, this particular policy, however, should be an integrated part of all development policy making. A minimum requirement should be that development organizations be aware of the fact that gender violence is not only an obstacle to development, but often also a consequence of development. They should see it as their moral obligation to at least prevent the latter, and contribute to development for women.

Gender violence as a consequence of development

Women are particularly vulnerable to 'the violence of development'[15]. Mainstream development policies on macro and micro level generally contribute to the oppression of women, particularly women who already belong to the poorest classes. The South is faced by the quandary of trying to protect women's human rights on the one hand and of introducing policies and programmes that undermine those rights on the other. Matsui[16] notes that, in common with many other women in the South, millions of Asian women suffer a threefold oppression:

1. Economic, political, and military control by the developed countries of the North.
2. As working-class women, oppression and exploitation by their own dictatorial governments and ruling classes.
3. Discrimination due to patriarchal tradition.

A case in point is the current increase in dowry murders. Many analyses have been made which all support Matsui's hypothesis that this increase is due to the cult of materialism, which is now widely acceptable, as a result of the modernization, economic development and consumer culture which envelop the whole of Indian society. This same cult of materialism has increased women's vulnerability to abuse by men competing for limited resources introduced into the local community from the outside through development projects. It has also reinforced gender blindness in government policies, such as turning a blind eye to large-scale prostitution and sex tourism, trafficking in child brides, commercialised marriage arrangements for the sake of increasing national income and serving the interests of powerful and wealthy elites[17].

Most literature I could find on the increase of gender violence due to modernization and development programmes deals with South-East Asia and the Pacific[18]. Howard[19] addresses the issue briefly for English-speaking sub-Saharan Africa. A difference with Asia is perhaps that there were less patriarchal societies in this part of the world in pre-colonial times. The effect of the introduction of Western ideology and the consolidation of nation states based on the Western model has been to deprive women of the political influence they seem to have had in many indigenous African societies[20]. Formally legislated equality cannot compensate for the erosion of such influence. Now communal norms are breaking down and women assume new freedom, men seem to use violence as a form of social control. Men are angry at women because they are no longer subservient.

A wife's assertiveness or her flirtations with autonomy have traditionally been accepted in many cultures as a reason for wife-beating and wife-battering. Surprisingly disproportionate vehemence and violent rage are seen as justified, because of the firm belief that the entire fabric of society would unravel if such wifely behaviour were countenanced[21]. Development policy aiming at the autonomy of women may therefore result in increased gender violence, at least in the short term.

There are other reasons for increased gender violence as a result of development. The tension, frustration and feeling of inadequacy due to the disruption of traditional economic processes through increasing landlessness and pauperization are often vented in assaults on wives, the most easily accessible victims. Because of this, traditional subservient and vulnerable positions of women are worsened, or traditional relatively independent positions are transformed into more vulnerable positions. Women are losing their significance in contributing to the family income in countries like Bangladesh, for instance, where mechanization in rice mills means fewer jobs for women. This can lead to a devaluation of women's worth in the eyes of men and consequently to gender violence[22].

Most explanations of the increase in gender violence in the context of development processes are traced to women's increased subordination in the structure of material production. The worsening situation of lack of property and resources denies women the ability to defend themselves. Ultimately, therefore, steps towards radical change in social and economic development programmes and projects become crucial for stemming gender violence. The Bodhgaya women in India who acquired land reportedly said: "We had tongues but could not speak. We had feet but could not walk. Now that we have land, we have the strength to speak and walk"[23].

For a full understanding of the relation between development and the occurrence of gender violence, therefore, we should also look for instances of a decrease in gender violence as a consequence of development and at the interplay between material and ideological factors. This understanding should lie at the basis of creating development policies and projects which are aimed at the reduction of gender violence in all its complexity, as a component of the empowerment of women.

Development and the promotion of women's human rights

Some guidelines for donors of development aid

On the occasion of the Seminar 'Calling for Change: International Strategies to End Violence Against Women' (The Hague, 6-9 June 1993), organized by the *Netherlands Ministry of Foreign Affairs* in cooperation with the United Nations Development Fund for Women (UNIFEM), the Netherlands Minister for Development Cooperation, Jan Pronk, promised to make a specific effort to integrate the issue of gender violence into the Netherlands development cooperation policy. He thereby took the results of the seminar (May 1993) organized by the Expert Group on Women and Development of the Development Assistance Committee (DAC) of the Organisation for Economic Cooperation and Development (OECD) to heart. The activities Pronk proposed to support are listed below in abridged form. The listing covers many suggestions made by others on other occasions and in a number of written documents to development agencies who are willing to support the struggle for the promotion of women's human rights[24].

1. *Research and data collection.* Research institutes and statistical offices should receive methodological and financial support for the collection of quantitative and qualitative data on the occurrence and causes of gender violence.

2. *Awareness raising.* For example, through supporting the monitoring of how women are portrayed and how stereotypes are perpetuated in educational programmes and the media, and supporting programmes presenting alternatives; and through gender training of the staff of the Dutch Ministry of Foreign Affairs, as well as consultants and partners from recipient countries.

3. *Empowering women through knowledge.* For example, by supporting advocacy initiatives to increase knowledge and understanding of rights, thus facilitating changes in attitudes and behaviour.

4. *Support to anti-violence projects.* For example, to women's shelters, psychological, legal and medical services, and police units run by and for women.

5. *Long-term support to local and international women's Non Governmental Organizations (NGOs).* For example, support for women's centres and documentation centres, and for exchange and cooperation between grassroots women's groups in the North and the South working on similar issues.

6. *Policy dialogue and government aid.* For example, support to national machineries and ministries, such as Health and Justice, for data collection, documentation of the many forms of gender-based violence, policy formulation and legal adjustments.

7. *Sensitivity to violence within bilateral projects.* For example, stimulation to obtain information on risks and occurrence of gender violence in development projects in various sectors, such as education, rural development, water and sanitation, health and family planning, urban planning and humanitarian aid.

8. *International instruments and United Nations activities.* For example, the use of the United Nations Declaration on the Elimination of Violence against

Women as a starting point for developing action in collaboration with recipient countries.

The role of health workers

While it is imperative that development programmes include the training of health workers to identify and possibly treat the consequences of gender violence in the form of physical and psychosomatic symptoms, a note of caution is in order here. Heise and Chapman[25] observe for the USA that today's emphasis on service marks a fundamental shift from fighting the causes of violence to treating its symptoms. Activists worry that the influx of professionally trained psychologists and social workers is redefining violence as a 'family relations problem', rather than as a crime perpetrated by men against women. In other parts of the world too, gender violence is now being recognized as a serious public health problem and addressed as such. The latest trend among health professionals is to focus in their diagnosis and treatment on the traumatic experiences of gender violence. Even though these trends are laudable in the sense that women's suffering due to gender violence is finally receiving the attention from health workers which was lacking in the past, the placing of this suffering within the realms of medicine and psychology should not be pushed too far.

The necessity for caution is well illustrated by the issue of female circumcision. Female circumcision has long been recognized as a health problem or as a problem of tradition. Although deplored as brutal, as torture and mutilation, it has, however, rarely been addressed as a crime or an act of violence[26]. This has only changed recently as the result of developments in conceptualizing gender violence and an ongoing Pan-African dialogue among women affected by the practice. The reconceptualization of female circumcision as a human rights issue has had consequences for the campaigns for eradication of the practice. This does not mean that a mere judicial approach to the problem will be effective. It is likely that only a joint human rights, health and development approach to female circumcision will slowly change women's affirming attitudes towards this practice.

This is just one example, perhaps the most well-known, which makes it clear that health professionals must make common cause with other disciplines in their care of victims of gender violence and endorse the link between physical and psychological recovery, and societal reparation and justice. The necessity for the endorsement of this link will be further illustrated in the following sections which focus on the identification of the psycho-socio-cultural complexity of symptoms resulting from gender violence and on the healing of these symptoms in the context of development.

The identification of invisible wounds

Even though it is now generally assumed that gender violence affects women's mental state in such a way that their capacity to contribute to development is reduced, very little systematic data is available on the mental health needs of women who have undergone or witnessed gender violence. Yet the psychological wounds resulting from gender violence may be much more severe and usually need much more time to heal than physical wounds.
The following story of Flavia from the Bombay Women's Centre, portrays the effects of battering on a woman's psyche.

> " In fact the body mends soon enough. Only the scars remain.... But the wounds inflicted upon the soul take much longer to heal. And each time I re-live these moments, they start bleeding all over again. The broken spirit has taken the longest to mend; the damage to the personality the most difficult to overcome"[27].

As a result of battering and other forms of gender violence, women may experience distress in the form of tension, fear, guilt, anger, anxiety, depression, humiliation, lowered self-esteem or confidence, and helplessness. Thus far, it has proven hard for outsiders like health and development workers and epidemiologists to diagnose these problems. Women often hide their problems behind a cloak of silence. We should not take this statement at face value, however. Women indeed often do not speak in a direct way about their emotional diseases, but this does not mean that they do not express their unease in other ways. If we want to learn more about forms of women's distress we must become sensitive to indigenous 'idioms of distress'. Abused women may, for instance, express their emotional problems in a somatic idiom, or they may become possessed by spirits.

Anthropological studies of mental illness in non-Western cultures have shown that the cross-cultural study of mental illness raises a number of problems of validity. In particular, the validity of the Western psychiatric diagnostic categories of 'depression' and 'anxiety' for non-Western cultures has been questioned[28]. Little is known yet of the validity for non-Western cultures of the diagnostic category known as 'post-traumatic stress disorder' (PTSD). This category has only recently come into vogue in Western psychiatry. Since there are indications that at least the main symptoms which characterize this category are universal, it seems appropriate to give a short resume of them. Knowledge of these symptoms and the ability to recognize them in trauma survivors will make us better able to understand why gender violence is an obstacle to development. The resume is extracted from the book by Herman on trauma and recovery[29]. Herman is an American psychiatrist who based her study on experiences of trauma survivors in Western societies.

Traumatic stress disorders

There is a spectrum of traumatic disorders, ranging from the effects of a single overwhelming event to the more complicated effects of prolonged trauma and repeated abuse. Examples of these disorders are the 'rape trauma syndrome', the 'battered woman syndrome', the 'post concentration camp syndrome' and the 'combat-related traumatic stress syndrome'.

The salient characteristic of a traumatic event is its power to inspire helplessness and terror. The many symptoms following the event (the symptoms of PTSD) fall into three main categories:

1. *Hyperarousal.* After a traumatic experience, the arousal of the autonomic nervous system continues unabated, resulting in: hyperalertness, vigilance for the return of danger, nightmares, psychosomatic complaints, generalized anxiety syndromes and specific fears, numerous types of sleep disturbance.
2. *Intrusion.* The traumatic moment becomes encoded in an abnormal form of memory, which breaks spontaneously into consciousness, both as flashbacks during waking states and as traumatic nightmares during sleep. Traumatic memories lack verbal narrative and context; rather, they are encoded in the form of vivid sensations and images. Because reliving a traumatic experience provokes such intense emotional distress, traumatized people go to great

lengths to avoid it. This too often results in a narrowing of consciousness, a withdrawal from engagement with others, and an impoverished life.

3. *Constriction*. The main characteristics are psychic numbing or paralysis of the mind. The constrictive symptoms of the traumatic neurosis apply not only to thought, memory and states of consciousness, however, but also to the entire field of purposeful action and initiative. In an attempt to create some sense of safety and to control their pervasive fear, traumatized people restrict their lives. Constrictive symptoms also interfere with anticipation and planning for the future. They narrow and deplete the quality of life and ultimately perpetuate the effects of trauma.

While in the aftermath of an experience of overwhelming danger, the two contradictory responses of intrusion and constriction establish an oscillating rhythm; with the passage of time, constrictive symptoms become the prominent feature of the PTSD. Since the significance of the constrictive symptoms lie in what is missing, they are not readily recognized, and their origins in a traumatic event are often lost.

Because post-traumatic symptoms are so persistent and so wide-ranging, they may be mistaken for enduring characteristics of the victim's personality. This is a costly error, for the person with unrecognized PTSD is condemned to a diminished life, tormented by memory and bounded by helplessness and fear.

Suicidality is one of the long-term effects of traumatic events. There is evidence that rape survivors suffer more from 'nervous breakdowns', suicidal thoughts and suicide attempts than survivors of any other crime.

People subjected to prolonged, repeated trauma develop an insidious, progressive form of post-traumatic stress disorder (the syndrome of chronic trauma) which invades and erodes the personality even further. Chronically traumatized people no longer have any baseline state of physical calm or comfort. Over time, they perceive their bodies as having turned against them. They begin to complain, not only of insomnia and agitation, but also of numerous types of somatic symptoms. They may become so accustomed to their condition that they no longer recognize the connection between their bodily distress symptoms and the climate of terror in which these symptoms were formed.

Protracted depression is the most common finding in virtually all clinical studies of chronically traumatized people. Every aspect of the experience of prolonged trauma works to aggravate depressive symptoms. The chronic hyperarousal and intrusive symptoms of PTSD fuse with the vegetative symptoms of depression, producing the survivor triad of insomnia, nightmares and psychosomatic complaints. This is often coupled with a tenacious suicidality.

The features of post-traumatic stress which become most exaggerated in chronically traumatized people are avoidance or constriction. This narrowing applies to every aspect of life - to thought, memories, emotions, sensations, activities and relationships. Thus, traumatic events not only violate the autonomy of the person at the level of basic bodily integrity and the level of psychological structures of the self, but they also have primary effects on the systems of attachment and meaning that link individual and community and damage relational life. They call into question basic human relationships; they breach the attachments of family, friendship, love and community; they shatter the construction of the self that is formed and sustained in relation to others; they undermine the belief systems that give meaning to human experience; and they violate the victim's faith in a natural or divine order and cast the victim into a state of existential crisis.

Psycho-socio-cultural healing

Stages of recovery in cultural perspective

Because the various traumatic syndromes have basic features in common, the recovery process also follows a common path. Herman distinguishes three fundamental stages of recovery: establishing safety, reconstructing the trauma story, and restoring the connection between survivors and community. Even though this threefold approach to healing in its generality may have some validity across cultures, the application of the Western effectuation of this approach in therapeutic practice may be unwarranted. Let us look at Herman's three stages one by one and make an initial attempt to test their validity cross-culturally. While doing so, I concentrate on the healing of survivors of organized (gender) violence.

1. *Safety.* In Western trauma therapies, safety is a precondition for further therapeutic action. What women perceive as a situation or place where they are safe, however, can differ per culture. While Western psychotherapists may succeed in giving a trauma survivor a feeling of safety in a therapeutic one-to-one

relationship, this may be much more difficult to realize with women of non-Western cultures. There, communal bonding between women may be much more effective. What is perceived as an acceptable sanctuary may also differ per culture. A more difficult problem is to discover how best to provide safety in situations where traditional cultural sanctions and sanctuaries for women have been lost, e.g. in a refugee camp where trauma survivors are in a limbo situation as far as sanctions and sanctuaries are concerned. And if safety cannot be guaranteed, such as in situations of ongoing conflict and violence where traumatization is a chronic affair, should we then conclude that any therapeutic action is useless?

2. *Reconstructing the trauma story.* The ordinary response to atrocities is to banish them from consciousness. The story of the traumatic event then surfaces not as a verbal narrative but in the form of symptoms; symptoms which are usually not recognized in all their complexity.

A major starting point of Western therapeutic therapies is that remembering and telling the truth about terrible events are prerequisites both for the restoration of the social order and for the healing of individual victims. The experience of many Western therapists who work in Western settings is that speaking the unspeakable leads to empowerment and that creative energy is released when the barriers of denial and repression are lifted.

There are risks involved, however, in encouraging women to speak the unspeakable. Women may not yet be able to cope with the truth and their symptoms may worsen. Another matter is that speaking *publicly* about one's knowledge of experienced atrocities is to invite the stigma which attaches to victims, a stigma which may result in ostracism and murder. If this is the case, a women might with good reason choose to let secrecy prevail or she might opt for suicide as a last escape from her suffering. What do therapists with Western therapeutic skills have to offer in these kinds of situations?

Despite the risks involved, women may nevertheless opt for speaking as a therapeutic act. As in the case of the *Testimonio* that is practised in Latin American conflict or post-conflict situations. Testimony can bridge the psychological and social recovery process. This observation leads us to the questioning of what Herman considers to be the third stage in the recovery process.

3. *Restoring the connection between survivors and community.* In the third and final stage of the healing process, the connection between survivors and community needs to be restored. Once the survivor has regained some basic trust in herself, she can start the process of selectively reconnecting with others. In the way Herman describes this process the individual survivor is the key actor.

This way of looking at the recovery process and its staging may not be very valid in non-Western cultures, particular in situations where people first of all suffer from the loss of their way of life, where the spiritual basis of their lives is undermined, where communities are shattered, and where human rights abuses are rampant. Here, therapists should make common cause with human rights activists and development workers. Furthermore, as therapists, they should be attentive to indigenous sources of support, meaning and healing which could be (re-)activated.

When people mourn the loss of their way of life, the phrase 'way of life' comprises not just economic and material necessities but also the basic value-premises which make an orderly and cooperative social life possible in the first place. It creates, furthermore, at least for many African peoples, not just the social world but the world: the order, whether natural or human, beyond the local community is seen as depending on the order within it. For a people with such a 'socio-centric' cosmology, being forced to flee their homes because of war or famine, or both, is an indication that something is wrong, not in the stars (as the etymology of the English word 'disaster' implies) but in society[30]. The reconstruction of the world, the repair of society, and the re-creation of the social bond, may therefore be a priority for trauma survivors who were used to live in a socio-centric cosmology. In that case, outside support in the form of comprehensive development programmes may be more beneficial for the healing process of the people concerned than interventions by Western trained trauma therapists. Western therapeutic models should be applied with caution, if applied at all.

Why early intervention may be beneficial in the long run

Many emergency aid and (mental) health workers find it remarkable how the overwhelming majority of people, particularly women, manage to cope in a traumatized society. Women are not per se more affected by the consequences of war as far as mental breakdown is concerned. The studies of Karam et al.[31] on the vulnerability of women in the Lebanese wars, for instance, indicate that both sexes are equally affected by the consequences of war in terms of depression and PTSD. Men do not seem to be more tolerant of the stresses of war, and they break down as frequently as women. Summerfield and Toser[32] found in a rural community study in Nicaragua, on the other hand, that 25% of men and 50% of women could merit a diagnosis of PTSD. Other studies have reported results of this order in war refugees and noted that women who had lost a child or spouse, or who had been raped, were particularly vulnerable to traumatic disorder. This does not necessarily mean, however, that women therefore cope less well than men in day to day affairs. The Comité de Defensa de los Derechos del Pueblo (CODEPU) found in a study of the effects of torture and political repression in a sample of Chilean families that, in contrast to males, women, and mothers in particular, had less difficulty in handling and coping with traumatic experiences. They seemed to have greater coping resources[33].

If relief agencies knew more about the mobilization of traditional coping patterns in times of crisis in a particular society, they could help facilitate, or at least not retard, these defences. Long-term studies, however, are necessary in order to determine how effective these defences are in the long run, particularly in a totally new environment where new sorts of stress (related to acculturation in a new society) may be awaiting refugees. The experiences of Jewish orphans after World War II and of Cambodian refugees in the USA, for instance, suggest that the nature of their reception may shape what happens over time, as much as the horrors from which they fled.

Thus far, we know little about the long-term medical and social effects of organized violence for the overwhelming majority of victims of organized violence who remain in or near the traumatized areas of their countries after such violence officially ends. We know much more, although still too little, about these effects on refugees who have fled from one Western country to another. What we do know is that a PTSD or a chronic trauma syndrome may develop a number of years after the traumatic event(s). And although PTSD is currently the centre of widespread public and scientific interest, many other psychiatric disorders are reported to be associated with war and other traumatic events. These include major depression, substance abuse, panic disorder, generalised anxiety, phobia, antisocial and other personality disorders, psychosis, childhood developmental problems, organic brain syndrome, and associated medical and social problems. Cumulative trauma can even result in personality disorders in the second and third generation, much like what happened to part of the generation which

survived the holocaust in Europe. Experience in Europe has shown that the long-term consequences of war traumas have long been underestimated.
Thus, we should not conclude too easily that people are coping well. Neither people themselves nor outsiders may have a good insight into what goes on under the surface. The question remains relevant as to what extent psychological numbing and devitalization, albeit operating under the surface, may compromise the efforts of terrorized communities to reorganize socially and economically, or to respond maximally to development projects.
Early intervention may prevent long-term negative effects on the health of people. A number of studies done in the West suggest that early intervention can prevent more serious long-term medical, psychological and psychiatric consequences. According to these studies, disclosing traumatic experiences is psychologically and physically beneficial. Inhibition of trauma-related thoughts or feelings requires physiological work serving as a cumulative stressor over time.
A case in point are the Korean women who were forced to function as comfort women in World War II. They had valid reasons to keep silent about their experiences in this capacity for so long. We have little information on how they have coped all these years. What is certain, however, is that the recent breaking of silence has helped them to release the stresses due to traumatic experiences in the past.

Support for long-term trauma recovery within the context of development
In the context of long-term trauma recovery the work of women activists from Croatia working in refugee camps has to be mentioned. One of their peace initiatives was the encouragement of the self-organization of women in the camps. The activists stress that basic work has first to be done in the camps, like communication between women and trust building, and that the specific needs of women victims of war have to be formulated before a concrete institutional system of support for long-term trauma recovery can be proposed. However, the basic principles which will have to underlie sensible support work can be pointed out from the start:

- Support has to be given by women, because only women can understand the deep crisis of the raped women.
- The work has to be done by NGOs to avoid possible misuse of the raped women for political aims.

- Support should be given to women's NGOs on the basis of detailed project proposals and clear selection criteria.
- Possible network of centres has to be decentralised and run by women only.
- Exchange of experiences between the women helping rape victims in different countries and direct support is necessary to build the needed network of volunteers and institutions as soon as possible. Help should be planned and organized on the long-term basis[34].

As far as former Yugoslavia is concerned, many initiatives have been taken by all sorts of organizations (governmental as well as non-governmental) to support the work with women victims of organized (gender) violence[35]. What has and will be developed in this area for former Yugoslavia, however, may not be applicable in other areas of the world. What is certain is that support by health workers to trauma victims in the South should be integrated in more comprehensive projects aimed at sustainable development; and furthermore, that an in-depth knowledge of the culture concerned is required for the establishment of priorities in psycho-social relief operations.

Conclusion

There is a general agreement in literature on gender violence that women's actions to stop gender violence and development programmes aimed at supporting these actions should be strengthened by research. Throughout my book[36] I have indicated what kind of research is necessary and formulated a number of (neglected) research themes and particular research questions. In common with others, I have furthermore stressed that the most difficult part of the urgently needed research concerns the psychological dimensions of gender violence.

One of the values of the anthropological approach to gender violence advanced in my book is its 'inside view' of what gender violence means for women, how they (try to) cope with it and its consequences, and where they fail in withstanding it. Anthropologists have pointed out that any research that can serve as a meaningful basis for worthwhile prevention and healing programmes must be of a certain type: action research, in which the findings are translated into programme intervention, and participatory research which involves members of the community in question in the research process. Some authors stress that the

necessary research should be done by and for women. Female anthropologists, for instance, should work with female informants. Another option is to involve the whole community, including, for example, male elders and religious leaders. It has been demonstrated in a number of countries that this latter type of research leads to community ownership of research findings and sustained participation in the resulting action.
Another requirement of the research is that it should, in many cases, be long-term, so that the effects of intervention programmes can be monitored and these programmes be adjusted accordingly over time. General guidelines for, for instance, intervention in the area of 'sexual violence and refugees' should be adapted to the particular socio-cultural contexts on the basis of long-term action and participatory research.

References

1. A longer version of this chapter was published before under the name of Linkages between development, human rights, health and gender violence. In: Richters, Annemiek, J.M. *Women, culture and violence - A development, health and human rights issue.* Women and Autonomy Series. Leiden: Women and Autonomy Centre. 1994. pp. 143 - 174.
2. Schuler, M. ed. *Freedom from violence - women's strategies from around the world*. New York: UNIFEM. 1992.
3. *International Herald Tribune* 1.7.1993.
4. Kerr, J. *Ours by right - women's rights as human rights*. London: Zed Books, 1993. p. 163.
5. Donnelly, J. The right to development - how to link human rights to development, In: Welch C.E. Jr. & R. I. Meltzer eds. *Human rights and development in Africa*. Albany, N.Y: State University of New York Press. 1984, pp. 261 - 285.
6. WHO, *Women, health and development.* Progress report by the Director General. Geneva: WHO. 1992. p. 33.
7. Sembène Ousmane in an interview with Van de Werk. In: Werk, J.K. van de, 'Vrouwen houden Afrika op de been', *Hervormd Nederland 49 (13), 1993. pp. 6- 9*. Translation by A.R.

8. Pietilä, H. & J. Vickers. *Making women matter*. London: Zed Books. 1990. pp. 45-72.
9. Shallat, L. Violations on trial. *Women's Health Journal* 3. pp. 45 - 51. 1993. p. 48.
10. Center for Women's Global Leadership. *Women's leadership institute report - Women, violence and human rights.* New Brunswick, N.J.: Douglas College, Rutger University. 1992. p. 23.
11. Buvenic and Yudelman 1989, referred to by Carillo, R. *Battered dreams - violence against women as an obstacle to development.* New York: UNIFEM. 1992. p. 12.
12. Pronk, J. Address on the occasion of the seminar *'Calling for chance: international strategies to end violence against women'*. June 6-9, 1993. The Haque. p. 13.
13. Mathangani, M. *Short study on violence against women in Kenya*, 1993.
14. *Linking women's global struggles to end violence.* Ottawa: Match International Centre. 1990.
15. Schrijvers, Joke. *The violence of 'development'.* Utrecht: International Books. 1993.
16. Matsui, Y. *Women's Asia.* London: Zed Books. (First published in Japanese) 1989 (1987).
17. Lopez, E.P. & J. El-Bushra. *Gender related violence - its scope and relevance.* Paper presented by the National Alliance of Women's Organisations (London) to the Overseas Development Administration. October 1992.
18. See e.g. Jahan, R. Hidden wounds, visible scars - violence against women in Bangladesh. In: Agarwal, B.(eds.) *Structures of patriarchy - state, community and household in modernising Asia.* New Delhi: Kali for Women, 1988. pp. 199-227. Korvinus B. *Grenzeloze sexuele uitbuiting. Vrouwenhandel - schending van de waardigheid en fundamentele mensenrechten van vrouwen.* Oegstgeest: Justitia et Pax. 1991.
19. Howard, R. Women's rights in English-speaking Sub-Saharan Africa. In: Welch, C.E. Jr. R.I. Meltzer. eds. *Human rights and development in Africa.* Albany, N.Y.: State University of New York Press. 1984. pp. 46 - 75.
20. Women's situation in Namibia, for instance, deteriorated sharply with the invasion of a colonialist regime. South Africa imposed a system which incorporated the restrictive traditions of earlier times as well as imposing more restrictions, so that such rights and safeguards which did exist were

abolished. In legal terms, women virtually became minors all their lives, with no legal rights. Regardless of their age, of whether they are married or not, women are legally always subject to the authority of men. Cleaver T. & M. Wallace. *Namibia women in war*. London: Zed Books. 1990. p. 78.
21. Brown, J.K. Introduction - definitions, assumptions, themes and issues. In: D.A. Counts et al., eds. *Sanction and sanctuary - cultural perspectives on the beating of wives.* Boulder, Col.: Westview Press. 1992. p. 3.
22. The Asian and Pacific Women's Resource Collection Network, *Asia and Pacific women's resource and action series health.* Kuala Lumpur: Asian and Pacific Development Centre. 1990. p. 195.
23. Quoted in Kelkar, G. Stopping the violence against women - fifteen years of activism. In: Schuler, M. *ibid.* p. 96.
24. Schuler gives a good and comprehensive overview of what needs to be done to confront the violence in women's lives in all its aspects: physical, social, economic, cultural and legal. Schuler, M. *ibid.* p. 96.
25. Heise, l. & J.R. Chapman. Reflections on a movement - the U.S. battle against women abuse. In: Schuler, M. *ibid.* pp. 227 - 257.
26. A'Haleem, A.M. Claiming our bodies and our rights - exploring female circumcision as an act of violence. In: Schuler, ibid. pp. 141 - 157.
27. Quoted in Asian and Pacific Women's Network, *ibid.* 1990. p. 176.
28. Richters, Annemiek J.M. *De medisch antropoloog als verteller en vertaler - met Hermes op reis in het land van de afgoden.* Heemstede: SMART. 1993/1991.
29. Herman, J.L. *Trauma and recovery: the aftermath of violence - from domestic abuse to political terror.* USA: Basic Books. 1992.
30. *Refugees returning home.* Report of the Symposium for the Horn of Africa on the social and economic aspects of mass voluntary return movements of refugees. Addis Ababa, 15 - 17 September 1992. Geneva: United Nations Research Institute for Social Development. 1993. p. 11.
31. Karam E.G. et. al. Vunerability of women in the Lebanese wars. *Al Raida 10.* Summer 1993. pp. 14 - 16.
32. Summerfield, D. & L. Toser. 'Low intensity' war and mental trauma in Nicaragua - a study in a rural community, *Medicine and War 7.* 1991. pp. 84 - 99.
33. CODEPU, The effects of torture and political repression in a sample of Chilean families. *Social Science & Medicine 28 (7).* 1989. pp. 735 - 741.
34. *Newsletter for Reproductive Rights.* January-March 1993. pp. 30-31.

35. In the Netherlands, for example, the recently established *Admira* Foundation has, at the request of the Dutch Ministry of Foreign Affairs, advised on the support the Netherlands could give to projects and organizations in former Yugoslavia directed at the reception of and help for women war victims. As a result a training project is in operation now.

36. Cf. note 1.

4. ROHINGYA REFUGEES IN BANGLADESH: THE DILEMMA'S OF SOCIAL PARITY

Marijke Wijnroks

Introduction

The nature of the refugee problem has changed greatly over the past few decades, both in extent and background of the problem. When UNHCR, the United Nations High Commissioner for Refugees, was established in 1951, the greatest part of the world's 2.5 million refugees was found in Europe, and most refugee flows could be linked with political persecution, in particular from communist eastern bloc countries. At present, in 1995, the total number of refugees is estimated around 25 million. Besides the increase in the absolute number of refugees, a major change in the nature of the refugee problem has occurred over the past years, being caused by a variety of factors and changes in the international political scene.

Long before the fall of the Berlin Wall, which symbolized the end of the Cold War era, sharpening of the North - South conflict had emerged as an important cause for international political unrest. Anti-colonial struggles in Africa forced millions of people to flee from their home countries. Similarly, military conflicts in Asia (e.g. Korea, Vietnam, Cambodia) and to a lesser extent in Latin America caused large flows of refugees in these parts of the world. Besides pure political persecution, related ills such as poverty and famine emerged as causes of refugee flows.

Nowadays, the greatest part of the world's millions refugees is concentrated in the South. The willingness of Northern countries to respond to the the current refugee crisis by absorbing more refugees is minimal. The incidence of violent conflicts directed against refugees has increased in several Western European countries and racism seems to gain more and more public support. As a probable response to this 'vox populi', many European countries have introduced new measures aimed at tightening the restrictions on entry. It should be realized however that abating the flow of asylum-seekers to Northern countries is not at all a solution to the mondial refugee problem. In contrast, the more barriers that are put up against refugees by the world's wealthier countries, the more this will add to refugee problems within poorer countries. It should be acknowledged that many of these countries have often accepted far greater number of refugees than much wealthier countries would ever allow in.

However, it is irrealistic to assume their full commitment in providing relief efforts that exclude their own population. Many countries in the South face major problems in feeding their own people, and it can not be denied that refugee influxes can bring additional economic, ecological and health problems, as well as security problems. As an example of the problems and dillema's that can arise due to the presence of large numbers of refugees in a severely impoverished region, I here like to discuss the influx of Burmese refugees into Bangladesh.

Rohingya refugees in Bangladesh

Since March 1991 an increasing number of Rohingyas, a Muslim ethnic minority group in Burma, crossed the boarder into Southeastern Bangladesh, fleeing religous and political persecution in their home country. By the end of 1991 the atrocities committed by the militaries were increasing and most of the rice harvest had been confiscated leaving the people without food, leading to a tremendous increase of the refugee influx. The number of refugees entering into Bangladesh peaked in February and March 1992 with 5,000 to 6,000 new arrivals daily, mounting up to over 260,000 refugees in May 1992. Most of the refugees came from poor families, who had not been able to 'buy' their security by bribing off the authorities.

The rather sudden influx of this large number of refugees imposed a serious pressure upon Bangladesh, a country with a high population pressure and overstretched resources. The Government of Bangladesh, initially well capable of responding to the emergency and reluctant to accept external support in order not to spoil the fragile diplomatic relations with its neighbour country, finally had to ask international assistance when the number of refugees became to high.

Within a short time, UNHCR and several national and international organizations were found providing relief in the refugee camps. Activities were carried out in the fields of sanitation and medical care, food distributions took place on a weekly basis. The food basket contained rice, lentils, oil and salt, providing approximately 2,150 kcal per person per day, which is well above recommended minimum standards. Nutritional rehabilitation centres were set up for malnourished children.

A nutritional survey, carried out in May 1992 by Helen Keller International - Bangladesh, revealed that the nutritional and health status of the refugees was dramatically poor[1] even compared to the high levels of undernutrition and morbidity that are 'normally' experienced in Bangladesh. A meeting of an expert panel was organized, comprising of representatives of all organizations working in the refugee camps, which concluded that intensifying the ongoing activities was justified. Appropriate measures were subsequently undertaken. The food basket was diversified with the addition of vegetables, dried fish, sugar and a ceral blend. Admission criteria for malnourished children into feeding centres were relaxed and it was decided to increase the capacity of the feeding centres so that other vulnerable groups, such as pregnant and lactating women, could be included as well. Although it took a long time before most of the recommended activities became effective, the health and nutritional situation of the Rohingya refugees improved spectacularly. A follow up survey, carried out in November 1992, showed that levels of morbidity and undernutrition had decreased tremendously to rates that were actually lower than found among the surrounding Bangladeshi population[2].

Considering the initial poor condition of the refugees, the number of deaths had been surprisingly low, and by the end of 1992 mortality rates in the refugee camps were even three times as low compared to Bangladeshi standards, as was informally confirmed by medical staff working in the camps.
Although living conditions in Bangladesh can hardly be considered as 'standard', they cannot be ignored when discussing relief activities in the Rohingya refugee camps. Bangladeh is one of the poorest countries in the world. It's high population density, at 777 inhabitants per square kilometer[3] one of the highest in the world, and the occurrence of recurrent natural disasters, such as floods and cyclones, only add to the problems of poverty. The poverty incidence, defined as

an energy intake of less than 2,122 kcal per person per day, was 84% in 1991, whereas 25 to 30% of the population was considered hard-core poor, with an intake of less than 1,800 kcal per person per day[4].

Most of the poor people have little variation in their diets, rice provides approximately 85% of the daily energy intake. Protein sources, such as lentils, fish and meat are consumed in small amounts. It is not surprising that the majority of the Bangladeshi population survives on rations that are far below the internationally recommended standards and that are grossly inadequate, both in terms of energy intake as in terms of micronutrient composition. The nutritional status of young children is extremely poor, some three quarter of underfive children suffers from chronic undernutrition, and between 10 and 15% of the rural children has a low weight for their height[5]. Deficiencies of micronutrients, such as Vitamin A, are widespread. Morbidity due to diarrhoea and respiratory tract infections is common throughout the year and mortality rates are high; life expectancy at birth is 56 years for men and 54 years for women[6]. Sanitory and medical facilities are generally inadequate, especially in rural areas.
Considering the 'normal' hardship living conditions in Bangladesh, it is hardly surprising that the initial warm welcome to the refugees faded when the number increased and the international assistance became more obvious. The local population suffered from several side effects that came along with the influx of refugees. Providing settlements for over 260,000 refugees, however crowded their living conditions were, further aggravated the permanently existing land pressure in densely populated Bangladesh. The collection of sufficient amounts of firewood became a serious problem, as well for the refugees as for the surrounding population. Road conditions deteriorated rapidly with the unusual heavy transports of relief items. Prices of some of the basic market commodities increased steeply and the risk of the outbreak of communicable diseases was a continuous threat.
The growing ill-feelings against the refugees even resulted in violent clashes between refugees and local inhabitants. Many Bangladeshis complained that the refugees had better living conditions than they themselves had. It was difficult to find viable counter arguments, considering that 84% of the Bangladeshi population lives below the poverty line and that mere survival is a daily struggle for most of them.

The Government of Bangladesh was faced with a difficult dilemma. Forced repatriation was not a favourable option, as well from a humanitarian point of view, as not to risk loosing international sympathy. On the other hand, the presence of a large number of refugees created internal pression and opposition. A rather irrealistic agreement for repatriation was signed between the Governments of Burma and Bangladesh, but took a long time before going into effect and soon came to a virtual standstill. Especially in the initial stage of the repatriation process, some of the returners apparently had been forced to sign for 'voluntary repatriation'.
The opposition against the presence of refugees gradually decreased when repatriation efforts became more obvious and even more after UNHCR had taken the important step of allocating part of their budget for relief and development activities in some of the surrounding villages.

Discussion

The situation described above is not new, nor unique. In Honduras and Mexico, in 1978-8 for example, refugees had better sanitation and drinking water facilities than did the surrounding population. Similarly, in Eastern Sudan in 1985, death reates among those who contracted cholera were one percent in the camps, compared to up to 20% in the surrounding villages[7]. Among local people it is the poor who bear the brunt, they may already be on the verge of destitution and hunger, and they are more vulnerable to the falling wages and rising food prices that typically accompany a large influx of refugees. With the increasing concentration of the refugees in the South, providing adequate care top refugee populations will be increasingly difficult, both from a practical as from an ethical point of view.

The Universal Declaration of Human Rights, the United Nations Charter that was signed in 1945, states that everyone has the right to life (Article 3) and affirms the fundamental right of everyone to be free from hunger (Article 11). While this confirms that refugee care is a basic human right and not charity, it should be kept in mind that the Charter of Human Rights applies to everyone of the world's 6 million citizens.

It is extremely complicated to design a well balanced refugee care policy, that does not compromize on the essentials of refugee care and at the same time does not create ill-feeling among the local population. The principle of 'social parity', aimed at bringing up refugees to a standard of living commensurate with the surrounding population, might seem reasonable.
However, considering the often wretched living conditions of people in these parts of the world where the majority of the refugees is concentrated, it appears unacceptable to apply these conditions as 'golden standard'. This is illustrated by the Bangladeshi case study, where applying the principle of social parity undoubtedly would have resulted in a massacre among the refugees.
Another possible approach is to design a broader developmental strategy, aimed at providing assistance to a whole region, instead of only to the confined refugee settlement areas. This options offers several advantages: integration of refugees into a society will be easier, the local population will experience less bad feelings towards the refugees and it can be expected that cooperation from local and national authorities will be better. However, the financial burden of such a strategy will be considerable.

Towards a solution...?

At present, UN agencies and most of the international organizations involved in refugee care depend almost entirely on fluctuating voluntary contributions from international donors. This encourages essentially ad hoc responses to individual crises and carries the risk of resources being taken away from one crisis as soon as the next crisis emerges. Since many of the Northern countries are presently promoting a regional solution to refugee problems and at the same time have decided to limit the numbers of refugees allowed within their boarders, they have left the burden of the refugee problems to the South. It seems justified that finding regional solutions to refugee problems includes the responsibility of Northern countries to allow adequate relief for both refugees as well as for regions with refugee concentrations, by guaranteeing sufficient and continuous financial support.

References

1. *Nutritional surveillance in the Rohingya refugee camps*. Draft report of the first round of data collection. Bangladesh, Dhaka: Helen Keller. International June 1992.
2. *Nutritional surveillance in the Rohingya refugee camps*. Report of the second round of data collection. Bangladesh, Dhaka: Helen Keller International. December 1992.
3. Government of Bangladesh. *Sensus 1991*. Bangladesh, Dhaka: Government of Bangladesh.
4. Government of Bangladesh, *1991 Statistical Yearbook*. Bangladesh, Dhaka: Government of Bangladesh.
5. Data obtained from the *Nutritional Surveillance Project for Disaster Preparedness and Prevention of Nutritional Blindness*. A nationwide surveillance system with bimonthly data collection in 20 sentinel points throughout Bangladesh by Helen Keller International. Bangladesh.
6. Government of Bangladesh, *1991 Statistical Yearbook*. Bangladesh, Dhaka: Government of Bangladesh.
7. Discussion at the symposium 'Responding to the Nutrition Crisis among Refugees: the Need for New Approaches', held in Oxford, UK, in March 1991. Quoted in: Keen David. *Refugees: rationing the right to life, the crisis in emergency relief*. London. 1992.

5. EXPERIENCES IN PARTICIPATORY TRAINING OF REFUGEES AS COMMUNITY HEALTH WORKERS

Jeanette Lekskes[1]

Introduction

This article refers to Hagadera refugee camp in Kenya which was established for Somali refugees in June 1992. Various organisations were responsible for delivering adequate care to the refugees. Soon after the first refugees arrived a participatory training programme was set up by Medecins sans Frontieres (MSF) to train refugees as Community Health Workers (CHWs).

The first part of the article examines aid organisations perceptions on refugee communities and the influence this has on community participation in health in a refugee camp. Refugee camps usually exist for many years and I will advocate a developmental approach in which activities are not only focused on health but also sectors such as education and agriculture are addressed with similar importance. Participation by refugees in decision making processes within the camps is essential in order to realise that refugees will take control over their own lives, and become less dependent from aid.

The second part of this article deals more specifically with the training programme in Kenya. Reasons for training refugees as community health workers are listed, and it will be make clear that the training curriculum was determined by a needs assessment carried out by refugees themselves. The general structure of this specific training programme, the teaching methodologies and recruitment of the refugees are discussed, and examples of the participatory training programme will be presented.

When a refugee camp is set up and established people often associate these activities with governmental, NGOs like MSF, Care, Oxfam and United Nations agencies such as UNHCR. However, without the participation of refugees as providers for health in a broader context, we could say that a refugee camp is not really established according to the Primary Health Care (PHC) concept.

Participation, I define here as that refugees have an active and essential role in defining and implementing activities related to health. Health in the widest sense could be seen as all factors which influence well-being. This article will give some ideas on how to work together with refugees. However, it does not imply that health is seen as the central and most important focus, but rather as a part of the development process in the camp. The article concludes with the recommendation that refugees should be trained as community health workers in a participatory way, whereby refugees establish services according to their needs, because they are the ones ultimately responsible for their own health.

Back-ground information

In Somalia in 1989 inter-clan fights broke out despite homogeneity of ethnicity, religion and language. Rebel armies organized along clan lines, overthrew president Mohammed Siad Barre in January 1991. Mogadishu, the capital of Somalia fell under the control of the United Somali Congress (USC), a group directly connected with the Hawiye clan. The USC split directly into competing factions under USC President Mohamed Ali Mahdi and USC General Mohamed Farah Aideed. Mogadishu and other parts of south and central Somalia slid into anarchy. The Somali National Movement (SNM) declared northwest Somalia independent and called it the Somaliland Republic in May 1991.
In 1992 the conditions in central and southern Somalia deteriorated steadily. Inter- clan fighting intensified in southern Somalia and increasing numbers of Somalis fled into Kenya and Ethiopia because of a combination of violence, anarchy and drought. An average of 900 refugees per day entered Kenya in 1992 producing a total number of 285.619 Somali refugees.
The influx required a massive emergency response. Eleven new refugee camps were established during 1992 in Kenya[2,3].

Hagadera refugee camp was opened in June 1992 and was situated in a rural area in Northern Kenya. About 15 kilometre from the camp was Dadaab, a small village. It was decided to develop a camp in this place because of borehole facilities. Initially, the camp was intended for 43,000 people. To make a space for the refugees to live, the area was cleared by a bulldozer.

Through a canalization system, water was provided by taps, there was no limit to the amount of drinking water available. A main hospital and intensive feeding centre were situated in the middle of the camp.
The lay out of the camp was as followed: There were 8 sections, each containing ten blocks. A block consisted of 120 families. In every section there was a service area with a health post, feeding centre and training/meeting room for CHWs. The refugees, who were mainly nomads, had to build their own houses from trees and sheeting which was provided. Food rations were distributed weekly according to family size.

Arrival of refugees

About 600-800 refugees a day arrived by trucks from the border. After registration by UNHCR and the allocation of a plot to each family, the refugees were medically screened. This included detection of very sick people and/or malnourished people, who were directly referred to the hospital. Pregnant women received an antenatal check card. Children were measured by walking under a stick of 1.15 cm height. If they could walk under the stick they were presumed to be under 5 years old and the arm circumference was measured to assess their nutritional status. According to the outcome they received a coloured card and were registered. Afterwards families received a cooking set, plastic sheeting, salt, rice, oil etc. They were taken to their plot, size 8 by 18 meters. About 80 % of the refugees were women and children.

Health care delivery

The central hospital was the highest referral level in the camp. It had an Out Patients Department and an In Patients Department. The hospital was managed by expatriate staff, Ministry of Health (MOH) staff from Kenya and refugees. A referral system was set up in which nurses and CHWs referred patients from the health post to the hospital. An intensive feeding centre was also situated in this area.

The main purpose of the health posts was to give medical care to the people close to where they lived. They were staffed by Kenyan Ministry of Health nurses and refugee personnel (CHWs). They mainly treated common illnesses.
Refugees who were identified and trained as CHWs were responsible for one block, preferably the block they were living in.

Perceptions of refugee communities

Nowadays it is common knowledge that health standards can only be improved if people become full partners to the health care providers. Often, however, health professionals tend to implement programmes or give advice about issues **they** think are important for the community, rather than to examine the concerns of the community itself.
The way in which a refugee community is perceived by the different organisations influences the level of community participation.
The term community can be interpreted in several ways:

1. In the health and development literature a community is defined as a group of people living in the same defined area, sharing the same basic values and organisations.
2. A community can also be defined as a group of people sharing the same basic interests. As people's interests can change from time to time it implies that the community members can change as well.
3. A third definition of communities is that of a target population or at risk group. This definition is rooted in the epidemiological view of a community[4].

Most refugee communities can fit in all the above mentioned definitions of a community in different periods of time. In the arrival stage of refugees definition number 3 seems most applicable, especially in emergency situations. In case refugees have become more settled definitions number 1 or 3 seem more appropriate. In the repatriation stage, the interest of people can change as some people go back home while others still can't. Definition number 2 will then be applicable.
Where a community is perceived as an at risk group only, it is likely that health professionals held to the idea that there is not much space for involvement of the

community: especially at the arrival stage the people are seen as vulnerable and disorientated. This perception still leads to medically-oriented emergency programmes with a top down approach. These are often set up by foreign NGOs[5,6]. This does not have to be the most appropriate way to 'deal' with refugees, however.

Exploration of community participation

The main question here concerns the nature of participation. Participation could occur within implementation of health activities and/or in decision making processes.

By participation in implementation of health activities the term is conceived as the mobilization of community resources, such as manpower, materials and creative capacities, in order to carry out health programmes. This often involves the incorporation of CHWs. Many problems could be dealt with by the involvement of these CHWs into health activities, rather than to search immediately for professional help. Moreover, self-reliance becomes enhanced by it. In this way there could also be more respect and understanding for the local and cultural ways of dealing with health and disease[7].The fear remains that CHWs are sometimes just used as cheap labourers.

Participation in decision-making for health is far less common than participation in the implementation of health activities. A reason for that might be the fact, that the first form of participation implicate the increase of people's control over the social, political, economic and environmental factors determining their health. In general, participation in decision-making means nothing more than that CHWs are chosen by their own community. That is the point where participation ends. The scope of the decisions in which communities may participate is usually narrow and health 'professionals' tend to keep in power. When there is participation in decision-making, the professional can less easily predict what the outcome of, for example, a needs assessment will be. It may include a reorientation from medical activities towards activities which include: agriculture, food, education, etc. For many medically orientated organisations, however, it is not acceptable to go beyond their field of professionalism.

Whenever an organisation makes an honest choice for a Comprehensive Primary Health Care programme this means that possibly activities beyond the field of health have to be included (one of the key elements in PHC is multi-sectoral collaboration).

Questions which are at stake here are:

- Is Comprehensive PHC applicable to a refugee community?
- To what extent is participation in implementation and decision-making applicable to a refugee community?

If we assume that refugee camps usually tend to continue for many years, a developmental approach is far more suitable than a medical emergency (top down) approach. I prefer to use the term developmental approach instead of Comprehensive PHC. Although in Comprehensive PHC we acknowledge the concept of multi-sectoral collaboration, where we try to link the health sector with other sectors, my opinion is that, even so, all issues in a PHC programme are situated around health. However, refugee communities and their specific problems are very complex. Therefore, it is not enough to see health as the central and most important focus. A developmental approach does include educational, political and other issues as well as health.

The issues are then interrelated and all of equal importance. Refugee community participation must be a part of the developmental approach. The participation should then not only be aimed at decreasing mortality and morbidity rates but also towards empowering these communities to take control over their own life which avoids also the possibility of dependency-relaters. It is advisable to gain community participation from the start of the project.

Before starting this work within the refugee setting, it is very important to explore the objectives of the different organisations in the camp, and what 'participation' actually means **to them**. Subsequently, it is important to assess who will benefit and what needs to be done to get a participatory process going in the project. It is essential to clarify these concepts, to see the different views people have and acknowledge their ideas about a feasible and valid involvement of the people and to combine ideas to a policy[8]. Through for example group discussions these aspects could be explored in the very early stage of the refugee camp and before any community based programme is initiated.

Reasons for training refugees as CHWs

Several reasons can be given why we train refugees as CHWs. Yet what benefit does the community at large receive ? A training programme could build on the knowledge, experience and expertise that exists among many refugee communities and use these skills at all stages of the health planning process. Refugees are able to give culturally sensitive care with accurate insight and as CHWs they could possibly find out which health needs exist and which issues are relevant to the community. CHWs who carry out home visits can get a better insight into what is actually happening in the camp and consequently advice the professionals. Generally, this could lead to a better understanding of the community and be a basis for starting community based programmes.

General structure of the training programme

All the above mentioned issues were taken into account and discussed before we started with the implementation of the training programme in Kenya.
The training programme was divided into two initial stages. The first stage of the training lasted for 7 days. After this training the CHWs worked for 14 days in their block to practice what they had learned. This was again followed by a second stage of training which lasted for 14 days.
The rationale of the first stage was to introduce the CHWs to the concept of preventive health care and to the role of the CHWs in their community. The introductory stage was also seen as a start off point in working together as a group, creating new community organizations and learning how the community could solve problems by themselves. The CHWs were taught methods how to conduct a needs assessment in the community .
After the training the CHWs worked in their blocks and conducted a needs assessment. Data on the demographic breakdown of the block were collected as well. The rationale of the second stage was to plan training and health activities according to the outcome of the collected qualitative data of the needs assessment. The results were discussed and further training was planned according to the outcome.

Teaching methodologies

All teaching was based on a participatory way of teaching. If one wishes to enhance participation it is important not to have a one way communication but rather a discussion where you listen to the people's priorities and needs. People learn more when they explore and do things by themselves. This will motivate them and give them more confidence. A participatory, or learner - centred approach, helps learners to take a greater control of their lives and develop their skills in problem solving.

In this approach trainers acknowledge that learners too have expertise and talent and that we build on that expertise. The more traditional way of teaching emphasises only the transfer of knowledge.

Especially, when working with refugees it is very important to acknowledge that they do have knowledge instead of seeing them as vulnerable. Refugees will then rediscover their strengths, so that they can take the initiative in planning and implementing their health services.

There were several other reasons for choosing this methodology. First of all the fact that most of the refugees had problems with concentration. This was because they were all bothered with so many other things and had to adapt to a new situation in their lives. Giving lectures would therefore not be a good method of teaching. Through discussions and problem solving techniques the refugees had the chance to express themselves, and come up with things which gave them more self confidence.

Role-playing and drama were used a lot, to let them express their emotions and difficulties in carrying out their work. As a substantial percentage of the CHWs were illiterate this method was the most appropriate.

Recruitment and selection of CHWs

When the refugees arrived the first section to be filled was the section A in the camp. When section A was full, recruitment of CHWs started. In every block some information was given about the organization of CHWs. A day was selected when people came together and the work of CHWs was discussed as well as the selection criteria. If a block-leader or elder was available he would help with the first selection of a group for interview. Afterwards interviews were held and 13 people were selected as CHWs. All community members of each block had finally to agree to the decision of selection. The following selection criteria were applied; The CHW must be a mature refugee resident in the camp, who is willing to share experiences and to learn from others.

General organisation of the CHWs

Each CHW was responsible for one block with 120 families, preferably the block he or she was living in. Training sessions were held with between 15 and 25 refugees, who worked and lived in the same sections. For example, the first group of CHWs all lived in section A and B. In this way it was easier for them to form a group. For each two sections there was one CHWs- coordinator.

There were equal numbers of male and female CHWs. Also an attempt was made to have a balance between younger and older CHWs. Preferably there would be an English speaking CHW in each group. CHWs from the same group met every morning. They started the day with role plays in which they were able to examine some of the difficulties the faced in their work. At the end of the week simple data collection was carried out. This included a report of what kind of action they had undertaken and the number of deaths, births etc in their specific block.

The training of the first group was carried out by myself and a translator. For the other 3 groups a CHW who had previously been trained (from the first group) carried out a part of the training under supervision. In total 72 CHWs were trained in this way.

We used many different training methods during the programme. The first two stages of the training programme I like to discuss in this article. An ongoing training programme was later carried out.

Examples of the first stage of training

Example 1

Health is often seen as the absence of disease. Other factors which could also influence the feeling of well being are often ignored. For example in a refugee community, CHWs will encounter a lot of mental problems due to the situation

the refugees are in. Therefore it is very important for the CHWs to have an insight into the broader perception of health in order to understand feelings of ill-health and well-being.
By drawing a line on the ground with on both extreme ends the terms good health and bad health we explored their ideas. This is also called a health continuum.

The first question we asked was: Where do you put yourself on the line NOW? Names were indicated on the line in the sand according to the answer.
The second question was: Where would you put yourself in a normal situation (if you are in Somalia). Again names were written down.
By questioning the difference between two instances where they put themselves, a intensive discussion was generated. People came up with all their difficulties being a refugee, far from home, missing relatives, relatives who were killed and how miserable they felt about this.
More than one hour was actually used to let the refugees express their feelings and emotions. Finally, a connection was made to the idea that health is not only a state of absence of disease and that different people could perceive it in different ways. This exercise helped CHWs to see the importance of feelings and emotions related to refugee status and related to ill-health.

Example 2
The 'pocket chart' was introduced as a tool for analyzing the needs and priorities as seen by the refugee community. By questioning and brainstorming about what the community might see as their needs, many facts and ideas came up for consideration. Brainstorming is used to generate quickly many ideas, but it does not give an explanation why those ideas are brought up.
For example the CHWs came up with:
* an ambulance to bring patients to hospital,
* tents for all refugees,
* better food distribution,
* more security in camp,
* creation of a market area

All these were written down and drawn on separate pieces of paper. Under each paper a small envelope was placed. CHWs received three different coloured papers numbered 1-3 in order to do a ranking. Participants were then asked to

vote which was their first, second and third priority by putting the cards in the envelope under the picture with the greatest priority.
Data collection was done directly after voting by collecting all cards from one envelope and putting them on the ground under the corresponding picture. In this way everyone present could see directly which issues were chosen as the most important ones.

Because CHWs were trained in this method themselves it was easier for them to go out to their community, to discuss the community's perceptions of health needs and prioritize them by using the pocket chart.The pocket chart could be used to find out perceptions of the community towards several issues like:
- "What services would you like to have here?"
- "What are the main problems in the refugee camp?"
- "What health issues would you like to know more about?"
- "Where would you like health education to take place?"

The voting cards can be replaced by stones, shells etc, according to the situation and the available items.

Examples of the second stage of training

Example 1

According to the needs assessment carried out by the CHWs, problems were the lack of food, no proper sanitation, stomach pain, and feeling of loneliness among younger refugees without family. These issues were further discussed and CHWs and refugees became for involved example in a sanitation programme. Stories from CHWs were used in the training to analyze the pros and cons of proposed solutions. By role-playing the different CHWs could try out a solution for the problem. Afterwards a discussion took place about which solution was the most appropriate in this story.

Example 2

CHWs had some problems in identifying root causes of problems and what they could do to prevent a disease.
The exercise we used to get round this problem was the following: we placed three sticks in the sand, each with a picture of either a CHW, a health post, or a

hospital doctor. All CHWs received another stick with a picture of a patient with a problem. For example a malnourished child, someone with cancer, eye disease, mental stress and other problems in the refugee camp. To indicate where the patient should be referred to each refugee was then asked to place the picture behind the CHWs, The health post or the doctor,and tell why that person was placed there. For example, a diarrhoea patient: you put it at first by the health worker who gives advice about oral rehydration, but also try to find out what the perceptions of the patient is towards diarrhoea, what causes it and how to prevent it.
The objective of this game was to make clear what are problems which could be prevented and how and to identify which problems have to be referred to others.

Problems encountered

After the initial training of the refugees it is very important to supervise their work and conduct ongoing training. Many NGOs set up a kind of initial training, but they do not realize that this is only a start. Reasons could be that a refugee camp is not seen as long term and therefore ongoing training is not appropriate.

Conclusion

Aid organisations should question their approach towards refugee communities. Is a short term relief approach where refugees are perceived as a vulnerable at-risk group, still applicable ?
Another approach, with a focus on long term development aid for refugees has been suggested. The participatory training of refugees as CHWs, where refugees are trained in finding out which health needs and issues are relevant to the community and how to solve their problems has been described in this article.
With this new perception in mind we can see refugee communities as active and dynamic, and together with refugees we could establish a refugee camp with services according to their needs. Only then refugees are not any longer dependent on aid organisations, but instead take care of their own responsibilities.

References

1. Many of the ideas given in the examples of the initial training stage were developed at the Health Education/Promotion for Primary Health Care Course in The Liverpool School of Tropical Medicine and were of great importance for me. I would like to thank also the people in the School of Tropical Medicine who gave their suggestions and comments.
2. U.S. Committee for Refugees. *World refugee survey.* Washington DC: U.S. Committee for Refugees. 1994.
3. UNHCR. *The state of the world's refugees, 1993. The challenge of protection.* GENEVA: UNHCR. 1993.
4. Rifkin, S. & F. Muller, W. Bichman. Primary Health Care: On measuring participation. *Soc.Sci.Med.* Vol 26. 1988. pp. 931-940.
5. Simmonds, S & C. Carlson, B. Dick. Community health education in refugee camps. *International Quarterly of Community Health Education.* Vol. 6 (1) 1985-1986. pp. 45 - 60.
6. Simmonds, S. & P. Vaughan, S. William Gunn. *Refugee community health care.* Oxford Medical Publications. Oxford; Oxford University Press. 1983.
7. Morley, D. & J. Rohde, G.Williams. *Practising health for all* Oxford Medical Publications. Oxford: Oxford University Press. 1983.
8. Srinivasan, Lyra. *Tools for community participation, a manual for training trainers in participatory techniques.* Prowwess/UNDP Technical Series.

6. HEALTH CARE FOR REFUGEES AND ASYLUM-SEEKERS IN THE NETHERLANDS: A PUBLIC HEALTH PERSPECTIVE

Loes H.M. van Willigen[1]

"Being a refugee means that you have many problems which you cannot tell anyone about, because no one will understand. There are people who say: Why do you come here? Our country is so small, what do you want here? If you tell them all you have experienced they don't believe you. All people have problems, but sometimes it is very bad. It just makes you ill. What am I to do, who can I ask for help, who can I talk to?" A woman refugee in the Netherlands[2].

Introduction

Since 1970 around 40,000 refugees have been settled in the Netherlands. In addition to this since 1990 about 30,000 - 50,000 persons request political asylum in this country every year. Among them more than 90 different nationalities have already been registered. Refugees and asylum-seekers have in common that they have felt forced to leave their native country. They have often experienced a sequence of traumatic events and serious stress before, during and after immigration, which sooner or later can lead to health problems. These health problems are generally manifested in so-called a-specific physical and psychological symptoms and social problems. Research on the victims of organised violence, such as victims of the Second World War or those of hijackings in the Netherlands, has shown that the timely recognition of medical complaints and the offer of adequate help may prevent the occurrence of more serious health problems later[3].

Seen in a public health perspective health promotion and prevention should form the backbone of refugee health care programs. The promotion of access to regular health care for refugees may also be seen in this perspective. Since 1980 the government in the Netherlands has developed a policy in refugee health care which is based on this view.

In what follows I will, proceeding from a discussion of experiences and research, describe the background of the health problems of refugees and asylum-seekers.

In doing so, I will further elucidate the importance of prevention, health promotion and the promotion of access of regular health care for the target group. I will then briefly describe the policy in the Netherlands with regard to the reception of refugees and asylum-seekers. In particular, I will describe the activities of the medical teams in the reception centres for refugees and asylum-seekers, of the Pharos Foundation for Refugee Health Care and other specific health care facilities for this target group. These activities in relation with the social situation of the target group will be discussed. I will finish this chapter by drawing conclusions and making recommendations with regard to refugee health care in a public health perspective.

Backgrounds of the health problems of refugees and asylum-seekers

In order to elucidate the problems of refugees and asylum-seekers I will start with a quotation from the book 'Primavera con una esquina rota' (damaged spring) by the Uruguayan author Mario Benedetti[4]:

> "When they break a political activist [...] and force his family to leave the country, they rend time, for these people, for the whole small clan, they give history a thorough shaking.
> Reorganising your life in exile is not starting from square one, as is so often claimed, it is starting from minus four, minus twenty or minus one hundred. Those who are unrelenting, who have earned their stripes in perpetrating cruelty, [...] it was they who inserted a gigantic parenthesis into society, a parenthesis which will undoubtedly one day be closed, when there is no one left to pick up the thread of the story."

As I have already mentioned, refugees and asylum-seekers have in common that they felt forced to leave their native country. Many of them suffered repressive violence in the form of imprisonment, torture, sexual violence, intimidation and house raids. Some were forced to go into hiding for long periods. Others fled because of civil war or other forms of political and/or social upheaval.
A working group which met in 1986 under the auspices of the WHO's Regional Office for Europe and the Ministry of Welfare, Health and Culture to consider the health risks of repressive violence, called the violation of fundamental human rights 'organised violence'. Organised violence is defined as: "The interhuman

infliction of significant, avoidable pain and suffering by an organised group according to a declared or implied strategy and/or system of ideas and attitudes. It comprises any violent action that is unacceptable by human standards and relates to the victim's feelings. Organised violence includes inter alia 'torture ..... cruel, inhuman or degrading treatment or punishment' as in article 5 of the UN Universal Declaration of Human Rights (1948)"[5].
Because forced immigration and exile are closely related to organised violence the working group concluded that refugees can be considered to be victims of organised violence. No distinction was made here between refugees and asylum-seekers. On the basis of experience and research it was also concluded that organised violence has to be considered as an important health hazard world-wide[6]. In what follows I will, for practical reasons, only make a distinction between refugees and asylum- seekers where this is relevant.

Practice and research have shown that in general refugees have experienced a sequence of forms of organized violence before arriving in their host country[7]. Political repression, arbitrary executions and torture are aimed at breaking the opposition to the dominant regime. By directing violence at individual persons, depicting them in the media as terrorists who threaten the welfare of society, or criminals who want to enrich themselves at the expense of others, and by isolating them during torture and detention, they get marginalised and there is a danger that they will experience the violence as individual. Political repression is, however, a means of preserving politically dictatorial systems and has an effect on both an individual and family level and on the level of society as a whole. Organised violence for political, religious or ethnical reasons goes further than killing or imprisoning and torturing individual persons. Threats and intimidation precede imprisonment, the individual is forced into hiding, relatives are arrested or 'disappear', an individual loses his/her job or is prevented from studying, neighbours can no longer be trusted and fear is dominant in the whole society or part of it. In a (civil) war innocent civilians often find themselves between two warring parties, who both accuse them of collaboration with the other side. Not only bombing and shooting but also imprisonment in concentration camps, arbitrary executions, sexual violence and forced displacement are forms of organised violence during (civil) wars. Both during political repression as in a (civil) war there exists a dominating atmosphere which has been described in

Latin American literature as 'ominous'[8]. Because of violence and the fear for it, families, or part of them, decide to fly as a form of physical and mental survival. Even during flight and temporary settlement in refugee-camps refugees may experience forms of violence and deprivation.

Arrival in the host country often means a fundamental crisis in the individual's existence. Latin American care providers, who themselves live in exile, described this crisis with the metaphor of the Janus face, that is, a head with two faces looking in opposite directions, which symbolises the beginning and the end:

> "One face looks to the past, expresses the breach, the loss, the separation, the homesickness, the mourning and the fragmentation of experiences. This can be experienced as a social death because of the impossibility of returning.
> The other face looks to the future, confronts the individual with an unknown environment, strange because of its social rules and impenetrable because of its language, full of real and imagined dangers, but also a place in which some relaxation is possible"[9].

Some authors speak of culture-shock in this connection, an experience that can cause fear, sadness and other emotional reactions[10]. Because of their contact with a new environment, a new culture with its own norms and rules, refugees experience a process of acculturation. Berry[11] has represented the seriousness of individual stress caused by this process in a diagram. The seriousness of the acculturative stress is dependent on such factors as personal characteristics, pre-migration experiences, education, cultural distance, the composition of the population in the host country (mono-ethnic versus multi-ethnic) and the possibilities for integration like getting education or employment. In many western countries refugees live either in isolation or in ghettos, marginalised from the indigenous population. Often refugees are unable to find employment, or are forced to do work which is below their level of education. On the other hand the host country often demands that they integrate in or adjust to the host society as quickly as possible[12]. Very often refugees lack relatives and a social network. Asylum-seekers must, in addition to this, obtain refugee status through a procedure which they often experience as traumatic. Here the interests of the host country and the asylum-seeker are opposed: the asylum-seeker wants rest, safety and support, the government of the host country first wants to see proof that the asylum-seeker has a right to these basic certainties[13]. In many countries, as in the

Netherlands, asylum-seekers are not allowed to work or study during the asylum-procedure.
In addition, refugees continue to be confronted by the repression in their native country through reports in the media and letters from home. Feelings of doubt, guilt and helplessness may be reinforced by positive or negative news.
Therefore it can be concluded that refugees go through a sequence of traumatic experiences and suffer serious stress not only before and during but also after their forced migration.

The (mental) health problems of refugees in relation to their backgrounds

For a timely recognition of refugees' medical problems it is important to gain insight into the nature of medical complaints and diagnoses which can be related to the forms of organised violence and acculturative stress which they have experienced. There is no consensus among the institutions which are concerned with the specific provision of assistance to the victims of torture and/or other forms of organised violence with regard to the diagnosis of the medical complaints of refugees[14]. The medical, and particularly the mental, complaints which result from traumatic stress are often included in the Post Traumatic Stress Disorder, a symptom cluster of psychological problems which is described in the DSM-III-R and DSM-IV[15] and which can occur as a result of various kinds of traumatic events, such as the sudden death of a relative, natural and man-made disasters. In general, these studies do not include the refugee's acculturation process. There are many publications on the medical, and particularly the psychosocial problems of refugees in relation to the acculturation process, but in general these ignore pre-immigration experiences[16].
For various reasons many care providers who are specialised in providing assistance to the victims of organised violence reject the Post Traumatic Stress Disorder as a diagnosis for their problems[17]. Generally speaking, for the victims the traumatic stress is not something of the past. Indeed, in many cases political repression in their native country continues, and the situation in exile is often also stressful. For this reason it is incorrect to speak of **post**-traumatic stress. It is claimed that the diagnostic manuals proceeds from a western concept and for this reason cannot be applied to non-western peoples because culture mediates the presentation of complaints[18].

In addition, the failure to diagnose Post Traumatic Stress Disorder could imply that these problems of the victims of organised violence may not be serious[19]. In this way diagnoses can contribute to the denial of the backgrounds of violence of refugees and therewith enhance their isolation.

The psychodynamic theories relating to coping with the consequences of traumatic experiences seem to offer more possibilities for describing the specific medical problems of refugees in relation to the violence they have undergone and acculturative stress.

Traumatic experiences are characterised by:[20]

1. Helplessness, i.e. the victim cannot influence his situation.
2. Acute dislocation of life, loss of existing certainties. The events do not fit into the ideas and expectations which the individual has about himself and his environment.
3. A profound feeling of uneasiness.

Coping with traumatic experiences is characterised by an alternating pattern of re-experiencing and avoidance. The goal of this process is, on the individual level, to regain control of his own existence and attribute meaning to the shocking experiences he has undergone. Regaining control can also be described as re-socialisation or integration[21]. The process of coping has been completed once the victim is no longer troubled by alternating re-experiencing and avoidance. However, the process may also stagnate or be extremely lengthy, resulting in psychiatric disorders, like a PTSD or other anxiety disorders or adaptation, somatization and depressive disorders. Re-experiencing and avoidance may be expressed in various a-specific physical and psychological problems, such as headache, muscle tension, gastro-intestinal complaints, general fatigue, anxiety, nightmares, preoccupation with the shocking events, disturbance of concentration, irritability and the tendency to isolate oneself[22]. Many times these symptoms can be seen as 'normal human reactions to abnormal inhumane situations', or as said, symptoms of a normal coping process of traumatic and stressful experiences. Generally the contents of these complaints directly relate to experienced traumatic events, like fear for uniforms, nightmares about persecution or headache attributed by the refugee to forms of torture like beatings on the head.

The most important factors which can influence the coping process and its symptomatology are: the extent to which the event was expected, childhood experiences or personality, including coping skills, the extent of support from a

social network and the cultural rules related to the expression of feelings. In connection with the last point I would like to refer to the many publications on cultural variations in 'idioms of distress'[23]. Given the diverse cultural backgrounds of refugees they will often express their distress in different ways.
Apart from the (mental)health problems as part of the coping process or consequence of the experience of traumatic events and serious stress, many refugees also present social problems which often are directly related to their social situation in the host country[24]. Examples are, housing problems, due to the obligation to share a house with unknown persons, even sometimes a political or ethnical opponent, financial problems, due to lengthy telephonecalls with relatives who stayed behind in the country of origin or family-problems, due to the changed roles of men and women in exile. These social problems again may cause a-specific somatic and psychological problems.

A public (mental) health perspective

It has already been said that there is a tendency, either conscious and/or unconscious, in countries where repression is dominant, but also in the host countries, to isolate the victims of organised violence and to deny its existence. This tendency, which is present in society as a whole as well as in the health care sector, is also called the 'conspiracy of silence'[25]: The avoidance of a confrontation with the effects of organised violence because they form a mirror which reflects a gruesome reality. This reality is liable to provoke feelings of guilt and/or complicity and helplessness with regard to the existence of organised violence. On the other hand there is also often the tendency, among the victims of organised violence, to avoid talking about the shocking experiences, and isolation is a symptom of the consequences of organised violence. In addition, xenophobia in the receiving society also plays a role for refugees which can, just like the 'conspiracy of silence' with regard to organised violence, be characterised as a 'fear of the unknown', or, as the author Elie Wiesel states[26]: "Fear of one's self".

The 'conspiracy of silence' was also dominant in western countries, including the Netherlands, after the Second World War with regard to war victims. Immediately after the end of the war government and society looked to the future. It was only to a (too) limited extent that attention was directed to the reception of, and provision of care to, the survivors of the concentration camps and the bombings, the resistance fighters and others who had suffered serious psychotraumas and whose social position was often very poor. One of the consequences of this has been that the problem of war victims has been raised to a specialist level: When society did direct attention to the consequences of war the confrontation was so shocking, and the experiences of the victims so repressed, that it appeared that only specialised centres could offer help.

The lesson that could be learned from the experiences with war victims, the victims of the hijackings in the Netherlands during the nineteen seventies and the Vietnam veterans in the USA, is that a timely recognition of the problems which result from war and organised violence may prevent serious medical consequences later. In addition, history has taught us that it is not only necessary for the medical world to recognise the medical problems of victims of organised violence, but that societal awareness is also of great importance for the prevention of serious consequences later. Professional care providers should not only take the multi-causality and complexity of refugees' problems into account, but they also should contribute to preventing their isolation and social marginalization (refer to annex a). For prevention combined action from the health care sector and social sectors in society, i.e. a public health approach, is required.

As stated, refugees have often undergone a sequence of experiences of traumatic events and serious stress before, during and after migration. Often, they present many aspecific somatic and mental complaints and social problems related to their backgrounds of violence and social situation in their host country. In order to cope with the experiences it is of great importance for the refugee to regain control over his existence and attribute meaning to what has happened. In general, preventive care should aim at supporting the refugee and, if necessary, at assisting him/her in regaining control of his/her own existence and the integration into the host country's society. Emphasis should be put on the identification and mobilisation of the coping capacities of refugees on individual and grouplevel. Medicalization of the health problems, which are caused by socio-economic, political or ethnic conflicts will have to be avoided as much as possible.
Refugees will not be able to cope with the consequences of violence and acculturation as long as they are in an unsafe and unstable situation. Initially, basic

needs, such as housing, food, safety and minimum privacy will have to be supplied. In addition to that, asylum-seekers will have to be given legal support and attendance for the good of the asylum-procedure. To prevent problems from increasing this procedure should be of short duration and above all understandable for the refugee.

On arrival in the host country, refugees will often present health problems that are related to the traumatic experiences they have undergone in their native countries and during flight and the stress caused by uprooting. In addition to that, refugees have frequently shown in practice that they have been neglecting their health, such as looking after their teeth, vaccinations and use of medicine. A medical examination, carried out immediately after arrival, would not just prevent the so-called imported diseases, such as tuberculosis and malaria, but it would also take away any worries the refugees might have regarding their health. Attention will have to be paid to the relation between the aspecific somatic and mental complaints and backgrounds (of violence). This would not only mean timely recognition of consequences of violence and uprooting, but also the acknowledgement of the backgrounds (of violence) and its consequences. Informing the patients about the relation between their health problems and their backgrounds, either individually or in groups, can prevent major problems in many of the refugees. The advantage of informing the patients in groups about the (normal) consequences of violence and uprooting is that the problems are being de-individualized. It might also lead refugees to organize self-help groups. Refugees themselves should be included in information and health education activities. Not only will this increase the self-confidence of the refugees involved, but the information can also be better geared to the needs of fellow countrymen and sufferers.

Most refugees will be unfamiliar with the structure of health care of the host - country and will not know what to expect of its various facilities. Information about those health facilities and the assistance offered can prevent frustration and distrust regarding assistance and will advance the integration into society.

In addition to that, the refugee should be supported in learning to find his/her way in the new society, to know the host country's norms and rules and to speak its language. For the integration process, and the reconstruction of a meaningful life, finding study-possibilities and employment is important. The access to education and the labourmarket for refugees should be promoted.

Refugees often worry about their relatives who were left behind. They will have to be informed about the possibilities of the reunification of families and relatives and they should be given assistance when applying for such a reunification.

For a timely recognition of health problems as a consequence of violence and acculturation, it is important that regular health care should have knowledge and expertise in this field. It could also be considered as prevention of serious later consequences, since the feeling of not being acknowledged can be prevented and the medicalization of problems can be avoided. There are some other reasons why access to regular health care should be made easier for refugees.
As long as regular health and welfare institutions are not (or not sufficiently) accessible, because of insufficient knowledge and/or interest, to the victims of organised violence who need medical and/or social and legal support, specific facilities will be necessary. They are necessary for the provision of care and assistance to those refugees who need specific attention and the improvement of expertise in this field. In addition, they have a symbolic value for the victims. The existence of specific institutions implies an acknowledgement of the problems of, and solidarity with, the target group, an acknowledgement and solidarity which is often not shown by society in general.
However, the existence of specific institutions also entails the risk that both the institutions and the target group will become isolated in society. Breaking through the conspiracy of silence then remains limited to a small group of solidary care providers. In other words, with specific health care facilities existing parallel to the regular health care there is a danger that the refugees will be even more socially isolated . The goal of the specific health care facilities will have to be to bridge the gap between the refugees and regular health care services. This means that the specific health care institutions' task is to assist refugees in such a way that they will regain control of their own existence and will be able to integrate into the host society, including regular health care. At the same time specific health care facilities should put their experiences and knowledge in the service of the improvement of accessability of regular health care for their target group. By this double track policy isolation and marginalization of the refugees in the host country's society could be prevented.
This double track policy has become even more urgent, since with the increasing number of refugees arriving in our country each year it has become unrealistic

that specific health care facilities would be able keeping up with the needs for specific care among this target group.

The Dutch policy on refugee health care

Since the beginning of the 1980s the Ministry of Welfare, Health and Cultural Affairs in this country has been responsible for the reception and support of invited refugees. This reception and support consists of two parts, Generally speaking, the invited refugees come to this country in groups. After arrival they remain in a reception centre belonging to the Ministry for about two months. There they receive, in addition to medical reception, language lessons, and a first introduction to Dutch society. They are then housed in one of the local municipalities. The Ministry subsidises the municipality in question to provide further support and language lessons during one and a half to two years. Volunteers are often involved in this work. Since 1987 around 500 refugees are invited to come and resettle in the Netherlands each year.

Since that same year till 1994 the Ministry of Welfare, Health and Cultural Affairs has been directly responsible for the reception of asylum-seekers[27]. During these years the reception-scheme has been changed various times and nowadays a semi-governmental body is responsible for the execution of the policy. These changes were deemed necessary in order to cope with the increasing number of asylum-seekers arriving in our country. However the philosophy about the medical reception has not been changed drastically since 1987. Asylum- seekers who have registered with and accepted by the immigration authorities at the border are generally housed in an investigation-centre for asylum-seekers for around 4 - 8 weeks, during which their application for asylum is studied by the Ministry of Justice. When the Ministry of Justice considers the application acceptable the asylum-seeker is resettled in an asylum-seekers centre. There he/she has to wait with (part of) his/her family till a permission to stay, as refugee or otherwise, has been granted and a municipality is offering housing. The whole asylum-procedure can take one to two years.

In the asylum-seekers centre a number of social and cultural activities are offered. Generally volunteers of the Dutch Refugee Council are involved in the support of asylum-seekers. Until asylum-seekers have obtained permission to remain in the Netherlands they are expected not to study or to find regular work.

However, gradually activities geared at the reinforcement of the refugees own abilities are introduced.
Refugees and asylum-seekers are insured for health care directly after arrival in our country or settlement in a investigation-centre. Since 1979 medical teams of the Ministry of Welfare, Health and Cultural Affairs has had the task of offering medical reception to invited refugees, and since 1987 this has applied to asylum-seekers as well[28]. The medical teams consist of doctors and nurses, supported by administrative staff, working in all the reception centres for invited refugees and asylum-seekers. Their task is to take preventive measures against tropical and other infectious diseases and they are responsible for the timely recognition of the consequences of violence, forced migration and uprooting, as well as other health problems. For this purpose a detailed anamnesis is taken which includes both physical and mental complaints and the underlying problems relating to violence and their family situation. Physical examinations are also possible if required. Nurses at the centres offer health education both individually and in group sessions, with the aid of printed and audio-visual material. If necessary the doctors carry out crisis intervention and they offer short-term care to refugees and asylum-seekers whose medical problems are related to violence in their native country and during the flight into exile, forced migration, uprooting and the often traumatic asylum-procedure in the host country. Regarding the asylum-seekers, the focus of the medical reception in the investigation-centres is laid on the prevention of infectious diseases, while in the asylum-seekers centres the emphasis is put more on health education activities and the prevention of consequences of violence and uprooting. The aim of the medical reception is to increase the accessibility of regular health care for the target group by functioning as a bridge to the regular health care institutions and by informing the GP and other primary health care workers in the municipality in which the refugee is housed of his health problems and their social and violence-related background, and giving them advice about further support and assistance. Discussion is going on regarding the transfer of the medical reception to the public health sector, the municipal health services (GGDs).
For those asylum-seekers who for psychological reasons cannot be maintained in a regular asylum-seekers centre, but do not need clinical psychiatric treatment, a special reception centre, the Abri, has been established. Mostly it concerns asylum-seekers with behaviour problems.

Originating from a merger between the former Social Psychiatric Service for Refugees, established in 1978, and part of the Refugee Health Care Centre[29], established in 1979, the Pharos Foundation for Refugee Health Care was created in 1993. The aim of this foundation is to promote the physical, mental and social wellbeing of refugees by contributing to the improvement of access to regular health care for them. The focus of the activities is laid on the support of regular health care services by providing advice, information, consultation, training, courses, the formation of local or regional networks and any other activities which may improve their knowledge and skills in health care for refugees. Refugees who are not adequately helped in regular health care can ask for consultation by the health care workers of Pharos. Also activities concerning health education, like prevention of female circumcision or Aids are developed. Methodologies are described and developed, research is initiated and documentation in this field collected. Internationally experiences are exchanged with comparable organisations abroad. Pharos works all over the country and has primary health care workers consisting of medical doctors, social workers and social nurses, divided over regional teams. A mental health care team, consisting of psychiatrists, psychotherapists and social psychiatric nurses is working more centralized. Staffmembers and documentalists are supporting the activities. The foundation cooperates and maintains contacts with many regular and specific health care and welfare institutes, like the institutes for the victims of Second World War, as well as with the Dutch Refugee Council, the refugee-organizations, pedagogic centres, etc. Philosophy behind these cooperations is to be complementary to activities of other organizations.

In 1994 a special pavilion of the Centrum '45, which provided clinical psychiatric care to victims of second world war, was opened for highly traumatized refugees who are in need of clinical psychiatric assistance. The Phoenix, a pavilion of the psychiatric clinic in Wolfheze, which since 1982 provided clinical psychiatric care for Vietnamese refugees, broadened its target group by accepting all nationalities among the refugees. A steering group, presided by the Pharos Foundation, coordinates the activities of all specific health care institutes and facilities for refugees.

Discussion

The centralized reception of invited refugees and asylum-seekers facilitates the timely identification of so-called imported diseases as well as the consequences on health of organized violence, forced migration and uprooting. Preventive measures can be taken, in the form of support and guidance regarding the coping process of the traumatic experiences and stress and health promotion activities can be started. A decentralized reception would hinder collective prevention and health promotion activities. However, it can be observed that with the increasing number of asylum-seekers arriving in our country the quality of the reception of this group has been diminished. The frequent moving from one centre to another, the lack of privacy, the diversity of nationalities per centre, the scarcity in meaningful activities, together with the lengthy asylum-procedure will have a negative effect on the wellbeing and functioning of the asylum-seekers. Very often there does not exist a multidisciplinary approach in the centres towards the problems of the asylum-seekers nor a shared view among the various disciplines involved on the interrelation of the problems with the situation in which the asylum-seekers are. Asylum-seekers and refugees hardly are involved in nor consulted about the health education activities; and activities geared at empowering the asylum-seekers are still too scarce. By the (too) lengthy stays of the asylum-seekers in the asylum-seekers centres apathy, passivity and hospitalization are often brought about. Therefore one could question if the current reception scheme in our country is not opposed to a public health approach of the health problems of asylum-seekers. Hopefully, the transference of the responsibility of the medical reception in the reception-centres of asylum-seekers to the GGD's creates more possibilities for a public health approach.

The possibilities for reunification of families are getting more limited the last years. Only recognized refugees are able to request familyreunification without any conditions. Refugees with a temporarily permission to stay, which currently is the largest group among the refugees, have to proof that they have a steady and sufficient income and housing before they are allowed to reunify with their family. However 60 % of the refugees in our country is without employment. Unemployment hinders familyreunification as well as integration into society, enhances the risk of isolation and has a negative effect on health. These factors should be taken into account in policies concerning immigration and integration.

Positive developments are to be recognized in the promotion of access to regular health care for refugees and asylum-seekers in our country. The requests to the Pharos Foundation from regular health care services for information, advice, consultation, trainings and courses are on the increase in the last years. This growing number of requests shows that there exists a willingness among care-providers in regular health care to improve their knowledge concerning health problems of refugees. However, equity in access to regular health care services means that refugees are able to find their way to and in the regular health care system and are adequately helped. Adequate help includes procedures which facilitates-access for a refugee to an institute, the right attitude and communication and knowledge of the careprovider about the influence of the backgrounds of violence, forced migration and acculturation as well as of the socio-cultural backgrounds on health, illness and illness-behaviour. This means that not only an individual care-provider in a regular health care institute should gain knowledge and expertise on this specific field, but that on all levels of the institute concerned policy should be designed for providing adequate care. There still are only a few (mental) health care institutions which recognize the fact that refugees permanently form part of our multicultural society, and therefore have started developing a policy aimed at this target group.

Besides, both specific and regular health care institutes are limited to health care in a stricter sense. They could play a more significant role in health promotion activities for refugees in a broader sense, like identifying sociopolitical factors influencing negatively refugees' health and health care as well as involving the target group in their activities.

And, finally, the growing expressions of xenophobia and racism in society obstructs any positive development in this field.

Conclusion

In general refugees have experienced a sequence of traumatic and serious stress caused by organized violence in their country of origin, forced migration and acculturation in the host country. Organized violence, forced migration and acculturation are compound concepts consisting of many factors which each can have a negative effect on health on the individual level. The tendency to deny the backgrounds of violence, the forced character of the migration and the social situation of refugees in the host country enhances the risk for refugees entering a vicious circle of isolation and social marginalization, which again has a negative effect on their health.

According to the WHO, health means an optimal physical, mental and social efficiency and well-being. Organized violence and acculturation appear to threaten all aspects of health, not only on the individual but also on family and group level. For this reason a public health approach, with emphasis on prevention, health promotion and the promotion of access to regular health care services, should form the backbone of refugee health care. Health promotion means more than information and health education. According to the WHO, in its policy "Health for All in the year 2000"[30], health promotion entails "the building of a healthy public policy, the creation of supportive environments, the strengthening of community actions, the development of personal skills and the reorientation of health services'. This means that health care sectors combined with other sectors in society should develop a policy aimed at the prevention of mayor long-term consequences of organized violence and acculturation on health. Refugees should be involved in the development and execution of health promotion activities. And regular health care services should reorient themselves towards the provision of adequate care for this new target group in our multicultural society.

Although the Dutch government has designed a policy in which the early identification of health problems among refugees and health education activities have a significant place, it can be observed that by the current restrictive measures towards the arrival of an increasing number of asylum-seekers prevention and health promotion activities during the reception phase of asylum-seekers have been endangered. The promotion of access of regular health care services for refugees shows more positive developments. Various (mental) health care institutes have started to reorient themselves towards this new target group in our multicultural society. Unfortunately, refugees themselves hardly are involved in the development of policies and prevention and health promotion activities till now.

For a real public health approach towards the health problems of refugees coherence should be created between the policies on health care, reception and integration and juridical/immigration procedures concerning refugees and asylum-seekers on national, regional and local level.

References

1. With special thanks to Ivan Wolffers and Sean Dézarts for their constructive comment.
2. Abravesh, S. *Vluchtelingenvrouw zijn is een creatief leven vol verdriet.* Utrecht: VON. 1990.
3. Bastiaans, J. *Psychosomatische gevolgen van onderdrukking en verzet.* Dissertatie Amsterdam. Amsterdam: Noord-Hollandse Uitgevers Mij. 1957. Keilson, H. *Sequentielle Traumatisierung bei Kindern.* Ferdinand Enke Verlag. 1979. Ploeg, H.M. van der. e.a. *Late gevolgen van gijzelingen. Een psychologisch onderzoek bij slachtoffers van gijzelingen in Nederland (1974-1977).* Lisse: Swets & Zeitlinger B.V. 1985. Dasberg, H. Social aspects of trauma following war, genocide and terror. In: *Health Hazards of Organized Violence.* Rijswijk: Ministry of Welfare, Health and Cultural Affairs. 1987. pp. 53-66.
4. Benedetti, M. *Beschadigde lente.* Amsterdam: Meulenhoff Nederland BV. 1985. (Translation from Spanish Fleur Bourgogne, translation Dutch-English by Robert Pool).
5. Geuns, H. van. The concept of organized violence. In: *Health Hazards of Organized Violence.* Rijswijk: Ministry of Welfare, Health and Cultural Affairs. 1987. pp. 7 - 9.
6. *Summary report of a working group on Health Hazard of Organized Violence.* Rijswijk: Ministry of Welfare, Health and Cultural Affairs. 1987.
7. Hondius, A.J.K. & L.H.M. van Willigen. *Vluchtelingen en Gezondheid, Deel II.* Lisse: Swets & Zeitlinger. 1992.
8. Lira, E. & D. Becker & MI. Castillo. Psicoterapia de victimas de repression politica bajo la dictadura. In: ILAS. *Derechos humanos: todo es segun el dolor con que se mira.* Santiago de Chile: Ilas. 1989. pp. 29-66.
9. Barudy, J. & D. Paez. Integracion critica: Meta de una terapia liberadora en el exilio Latinoamericano. In: *Asi Buscamos Rehacernos, Repression, Exilio, Trabajo Psico-Social.* COLAT/CELADEC. Diciembre 1980.
10. Garza-Guerrero, A.C. Culture shock: its mourning and the vicissitudes of identity. *Journal of the American Psychoanalytic Association.* 22. 1974. pp. 408-429.
11. Berry, J.W. Acculturation and psychological adaptation among refugees. In: Miserez Diana (ed.) *Refugees - the trauma of exile; The humanitarian role of Red Cross and Red Crescent.* Dordrecht: Martinus Nijhoff Publishers. 1988.

pp. 97-110. Williams, C.L. & J.W. Primary prevention of acculturative stress among refugees; Application of psychological theory and practice. *American Psychogist*. Vol 46, 6. 1991. pp. 632-641.

12. Waelen, W.J.M. & A.A.M. Postel. *Vluchtelingen: een vooronderzoek naar het integratieproces*. Nijmegen: Onderzoeks- en Adviesbureau Geerts. 1991.
13. Emminghaus, W.B. From first aid in emergencies to intercultural encounters. In: Miserez, Diana. *ibid*. pp. 111 - 131.
14. Willigen L.H.M. & A.J.K. Hondius. *Vluchtelingen en Gezondheid.* Deel I. Lisse: Swets & Zeitlinger. 1992.
15. American Psychiatric Association. *Diagnostic and Statistical Manual of Mental Disorders*. 3rd revised edition, 4th edition. Washington DC: American Psychiatric Association. 1987, 1994.
16. Willigen, L.J.M. & A.J.K. Hondius *ibid.*
17. *Synthesis of conclusions. First World Meeting of Medical and Psychosocial Centres specialized in the treatment of victims of organized violence in Paris 1987.* Paris/Rijswijk. 1988.
18. Kleber, R.J. & D. Brom & P.B. Defares. *Traumatische ervaringen, gevolgen en verwerking*. Lisse: Swets en Zeitlinger B.V. 1986.
19. Lansen, J. Een kritische opinie over het begrip posttraumatische stressstoornis. *ICODO-info 89-4/90-1*. pp. 11 - 18.
20. Kleber, R.J. & D. Brom & P.B. Defares. *ibid.* American Psychiatric Association. *ibid*. 1994.
21. Begemann, F.A. *Reacties op geweld*. Utrecht: Stichting ICODO. Okt. 1987.
22. Hondius, A.J.K. & L.H.M. van Willigen. *ibid.*
23. Westermeyer, J. Psychiatric diagnoses across cultural boundaries. *Am J Psychiatry* 142 (7). 1985. pp. 798 - 805. Kirmayer, L.J. Cultural variations in the response to psychiatric disorders and emotional distress. Soc Sci Med 1989. 29 (3). pp. 327-339.
24. Hondius, A.J.K. & L.H.M. van Willigen. *ibid.*
25. Danieli, Y. Psychotherapists' participation in the conspiracy of silence about the Holocaust. *Psychoanalytic psychology* 1, 1984. pp. 23 - 43. Bustos, E. Dealing with the unbearable. Reactions of therapists and therapeutic institutions to survivors of torture. In: Suedfield Peter (Ed). *Psychology and torture*. New York: Hemisphere. 1990.
26. Wiesel, E. *Volkskrant*. August 1991.

27. In September 1994 the responsibility for the reception of asylum-seekers, including the medical reception was transferred to the Ministry of Justice.
28. Since 1992 the medical teams in the reception centres for asylum-seekers fall under the responsibility of the semi-governmental body, the Central Reception of Asylum-seekers (COA).
29. The former Refugee Health Care Centre was part of the Ministry of Welfare, Health and Cultural Affairs. the medical reception in the reception centres for invited refugees and asylum-seekers fell under the responsibility of this Centre till 1992.
30. *Targets for health for all.* Copenhagen: World Health Organization, Regional Office for Europe. 1985

ANNEX A THE VICIOUS CIRCLE OF ISOLATION OF REFUGEES AND ASYLUM-SEEKERS IN SOCIETY AND IN THE REGULAR HEALTH CARE SECTOR IN THE HOST COUNTRY

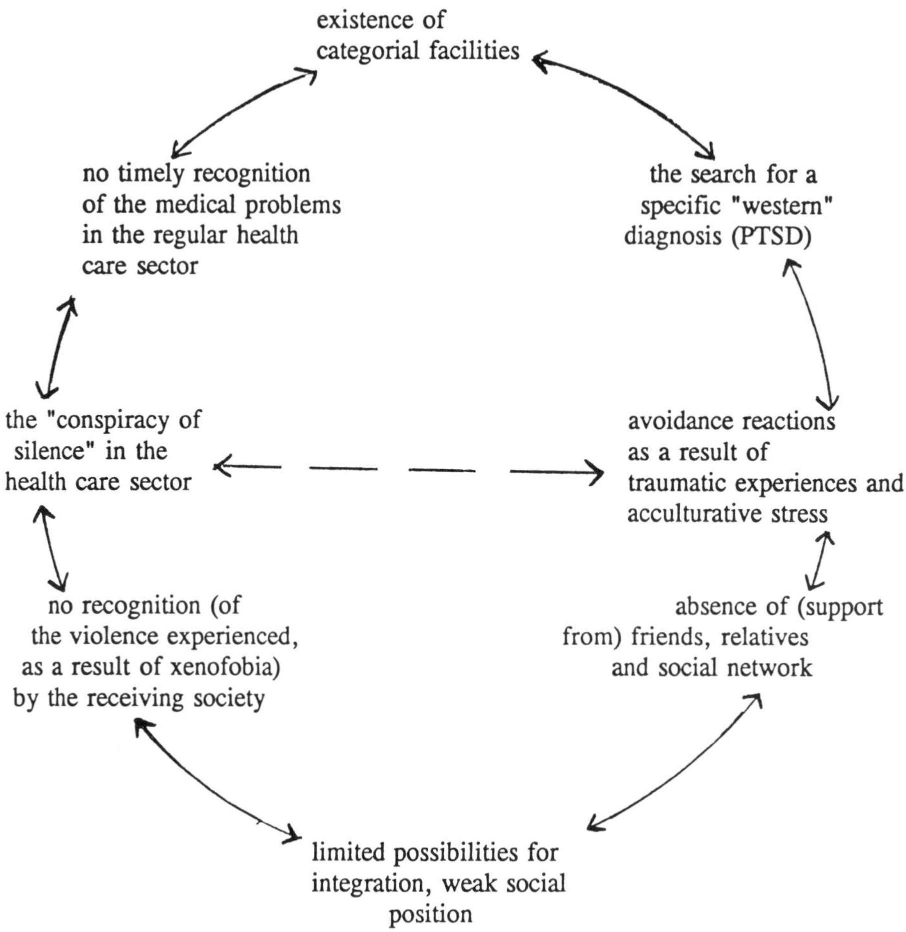

LIST OF ABBREVIATIONS

CHWs	Community Health Worker
COA	Central Reception of Asylum-seekers
DAC	Development Assistance Committee
DIA	Dutch Interchurch Aid
DSM	Diagnostic & Statistical Manual for Mental Disorders
FLS	Nairobi Forward Looking Strategies for the Advancement of Women: equality, development and peace. 1985
GGD	Dutch Municipal Health Services
ICCO	Interchurch Organization for Development Cooperation
IMF	International Monetary Fund
IRTC	International Rehabilitation Council for Torture Victims
MOH	Ministry of Health
Memisa	Foundation Memisa Medicus Mundi
MSF	Medecins Sans Frontieres
NCO	National Committee For Development Education
NGO(s)	Non Governmental Organisation(s)
OECD	Organisation for Economic Cooperation and Development
PAHO	Panamerican Health Organization

PHC	Primary Health Care
PTSD	Post-Traumatic Stress Disorder
RAWOO	The Council of Advice on Scientific Research in Developing Countries
SNM	Somali National Movement
UN	United Nations
UNHCR	United Nations High Commissioner for Refugees
UNICEF	United Nations Children's Fund
USC	United Somali Congress
WHO	World Health Organisation

LIST OF CONTRIBUTORS

Anica Mikus Kos

Dr. Anica Mikus Kos is a Slovenian Consultant Child Psychiatrist. After 4 years of being the Head of the Department of Child Psychiatry at the University Paediatric Clinic in Ljubljana, she became a senior researcher at the Institute of Sociology, University of Ljubljana. The last sixteen years she worked as the Director of the Counselling Centre for Children, Adolescents and Parents in Ljubljana. She devoted her professional efforts mainly to the development of community and population oriented models of child mental health protection with special interest in the introduction of mental health principles in primary and secondary schools. The last three years she has also been involved in psychosocial help to refugees from Bosnia and Herzogovina living in Slovenia. Currently she is the Vice-President of the European Society for Child and Adolescent Psychiatry, she is a member of the National Commission for Medical Ethics, and works as a UNICEF's consultant for psycho-social programmes. Besides, she holds the position of National WHO coordinator for Child mental health and finally she is also the President of the Slovene Foundation.

Anke van der Kwaak

Anke van der Kwaak is an anthropologist who works mainly in the field of health care, human rights and gender issues. The region of her special interest is the Horn of Africa. There she has been involved in e.g. research within Primary Health Care Programmes, gender issues and election monitoring. Since 1990 she has worked for Amnesty International as a country-specialist on the Horn of Africa/Somalia. In 1993 she became research coordinator of the Women and Autonomy Centre (VENA) of the Institute of Cultural Studies of Leiden University. Till the end of 1995 she worked there as a researcher and an gender trainer. Besides, she was involved in consultancies in the field of traffic in women, incentives and reproductive health, violence against women, gender and infrastructure and emergency aid.

Since 1992 she has been lecturer in 'Culture and Health' at the Department of Social Medicine, Free University of Amsterdam. She is a member of the Working Group on Gender, Conflict and Development of the Council for Gender Experts for Development Cooperation.

Jeanette Lekskes

Jeanette Lekses is a nurse and trainer. From 1990 till 1992 she was working with displaced people in Sudan and refugees in Kenya. She was involved in setting up participatory training programmes for health workers in these camps. In 1992 she successfully attended the course 'Health Education promotion for PHC' at the Liverpool School of Tropical Medicine. In 1993 she took her Nursing Tutor Degree, and in 1995 she obtained a Masters in Development Studies at the Centre For Development Studies, University of Leeds, United Kingdom. At present she is a free-lance consultant and lecturer in health education.

Annemiek J.M. Richters

Annemiek Richters has a multi-disciplinary training in medicine, anthropology, sociology and philosophy. As a physician she worked in several health care sectors in the Netherlands as well as abroad. As a social scientist she did field-work in a number of countries, and was appointed as a lecturer and researcher at different university departments. The subject of her doctoral thesis (1991) is 'The medical anthropologist as narrator and translator'. She wrote the book 'Women, culture and violence' during her stay at The Women and Autonomy Centre (VENA) of Leiden University. In 1994 she spent 8 months in Sarajevo as 'traumatic stress programme developer' for MSF-Holland. Since April 1995 she holds the Henny Verhagen Chair for Women-and-health-care at The University Medical Centre of Leiden University. Her present interest is 'women, culture and health with a special focus on 'sexuality and violence' and 'heart and soul'.

Loes van Willigen

Loes van Willigen received her medical degree in 1972, and she worked as a general practitioner in Edam, the Netherlands. In 1982 she joined the former Refugee Health Care Centre, and was mainly concerned with the care for Latin American and women refugees. In 1985 she became the director of this centre. Since 1994 she has been the Medical Director of the Pharos Foundation for Refugee Health Care, originating from a merger between the Social Psychiatric Service for Refugees and a part of the former Refugee Health Care Centre.
In 1992 she received a doctorate on her dissertation 'Refugees and health. Theoretical Considerations regarding the medical complaints of refugees in Primary Health Care'. She was the acting Secretary General of the International Society for Health and Human Rights, founded in 1993 of which she is now the Honourary President. Since 199O she coordinates on request of the Regional Office for Europe of the WHO the Advisory Group on 'the health situation of refugees and victims of organized violence'. She also is a member of the International Society for Traumatic Stress Studies and the International Association for the Study of Forced Migration.

Ivan Wolffers

Ivan Wolffers is a medical doctor, a researcher, a writer and a publicist. Since 1989 he holds a chair in 'Health care in developing countries' at the Department of Social Medicine of the Free University of Amsterdam. He graduated as a general physician, and worked in health education and primary health care. In 1987 he received a doctorate in medical anthropology on the thesis 'Changing Traditions in Health Care (Sri Lanka)'. In 1990 he founded the publication series 'Primary Health Care in Practice'. Since 1990 he has been a member of the RAWOO, the Council of Advice on Scientific Research in Developing Countries for the Department of International Cooperation (DGIS) of the Ministry of Foreign Affairs.
Since 1978 he has been involved in many missions and consultancies concerning many different topics in various countries and continents in the world. His main interest are pharmaceuticals, Primary Health Care and participatory research.

Besides, he is a well-known national and international publicist. In the last years he has been particularly interested and involved in altering the image of Aids.

Marijke Wijnroks

Marijke Wijnroks is a medical doctor, who got a her special training in tropical health and medicine from the Prins Leopold Institute for Tropical Health and Medicine, Antwerp, Belgium. From 1987 up to 1991 she worked for Medicins Sans Frontieres Holland. She was involved in basic medical care in settlements for displaced people in Southern Sudan. After that she became the medical coordinator of PHC project in Uganda, which included the medical care in a camp of Sudanese refugees. In 1991 she was based in the Netherlands and concerned with the design of guidelines for intervention in epidemics in refugee camps. From 1991 - 1993 she worked as a technical advisor in a nutritional surveillance project of Helen Keller International in Dhaka, Bangladesh. One of her tasks involved the coordination of the surveillance project in Rohingya refugee camps. At present she works as a technical advisor in to Community Based Health Care Projects of the Panamerican Health Organization (PAHO/-WHO) in El Salvador.